Better X-Ray Interpretation

Kathy J. Scheffer, RN
Richard S. Tobin, MD

D0967424

Springhouse Corporation
Springhouse, Pennsylvania

Staff

Executive Director
Matthew Cahill

Editorial Director
Patricia Schull, RN, MSN

Clinical Manager
Judith Schilling McCann, RN, MSN

Art Director
John Hubbard

Managing Editor
A.T. McPhee, RN, BSN

Senior Editor
Michael Lear-Olimpi

Clinical Editor
Ann Barrow, RN, MSN

Copy Editors
Cynthia C. Breuninger (manager), Christine Cunniffe, Brenna Mayer, Christina P. Ponzcek

Designers
Arlene Putterman (senior associate art director), Mary Ludwicki (book designer), Elaine Ezrow

Typography
Diane E. Paluba (manager), Joyce Rossi Biletz, Phyllis Marron, Valerie Rosenberger

Manufacturing
Deborah Meiris (director), Pat Dorshaw (manager), Anna Brindisi, T.A. Landis

Production Coordinator
Margaret A. Rastiello

Editorial Assistants
Beverly Lane, Mary Madden, Jeanne Napier

℞ A member of the Reed Elsevier plc group

Library of Congress Cataloging-in-Publication Data
Scheffer, Kathy J.
  Better X-ray interpretation / Kathy J. Scheffer, Richard S. Tobin.
      p. cm.
Includes index.
1. Radiography, Medical — Handbooks, manuals, etc. I. Tobin, Richard S. II. Title.
[DNLM: 1. Radiography—handbooks. 2. Radiography—nurses' instruction. WN 39 S317b 1996]
RC78.S186 1996
616.07'572—dc20
DNLM/DLC   96-30285
ISBN 0-87434-868-4 (alk. paper)   CIP

Contents

Acknowledgments

We'd like to recognize all the people who helped with this book. As we learned along the way, writing a book is a huge undertaking that cannot be accomplished without help — lots of it.

Our gratitude and acknowledgement go to Sonya Zwenger-Miller, RN, who contributed to the project her knowledge, organizational and technical skills, and friendship.

To the radiologists who found cases, wrote excerpts, edited, and encouraged us, we say thank you. We extend special thanks to Dr. Don Rose, Dr. Frank Wessbecher, Dr. Drew Deutsch, and Dr. Tom Keskey for their knowledge, help, and use of diagnostic images.

Our thanks also go to the radiologic technologists who found book-quality images, offered us encouragement, and expressed interest in this project. We particularly appreciated the efforts of William Roberts, RT, CVT, who copied all the films for reproduction. Thanks, too, to Chris Willard of St. Joseph's Hospital in Tacoma, Washington, for reproduction of images.

We wish to recognize the administration and staff of Tacoma General Hospital for lending computer equipment, technical assistance, and support services.

To the staff of Springhouse Corporation, who helped get us started, put their trust in our abilities, listened to our concerns, and helped bring the project to completion, we owe our gratitude.

Finally, to our families, who put up with deadlines and tired, absentee spouses and parents — yet kept the home fires burning — we express our heartfelt thanks and appreciation. And finally, to answer their often-asked question of whether we're done yet, we say: Yes, we made it!

Kathy J. Scheffer, RN, and Richard S. Tobin, MD

Preface

One hundred years ago, Wilhelm Roentgen's discovery of a mysterious new kind of ray, dubbed the "X" ray, created a worldwide sensation. Within a year, about 50 books and 1,000 papers had been published on X-rays. Since then, the body of written works on radiology has mushroomed as fast as new technologies have exploded onto the diagnostic scene. *Better X-Ray Interpretation* is our contribution.

Quality care on the cutting edge
Once offering only X-rays—and strictly as a diagnostic tool—radiology has evolved into a cutting-edge discipline with diverse applications. Besides allowing clinicians to look inside the body without invading it, radiology now has therapeutic uses.

A poor understanding of radiology can put health care professionals and their patients at a clear disadvantage. Suppose, for instance, you're the one who's responsible for explaining magnetic resonance imaging (MRI) to a patient scheduled for an MRI scan. You need to explain how the procedure is performed, what kind of preparation he'll need, and whether there are potential risks.

And consider this: In some clinical settings, a nurse or resident is often the first person to view a patient's X-ray. If you found yourself in this position, would you know enough about X-ray images to examine the film for clues to your patient's condition?

Our primary objective in writing *Better X-Ray Interpretation* was simple: to provide nurses, residents, nurse practitioners, physician assistants, and other allied health professionals with an easy-to-read guide to assessing radiographic images. To further that aim, we strove to present the information in the clearest possible way.

Greater understanding means better care

Our ultimate goal, of course, was to improve patient care. How can greater understanding of radiology help you achieve that goal? Let's say your patient has just had a triple-lumen subclavian catheter inserted, with correct catheter placement confirmed by a chest X-ray. Shortly after viewing the X-ray, you return to the patient's room to find him sitting upright, complaining of shortness of breath and chest pain. A vital sign check tells you he's tachypneic and tachycardic. In most instances, these signs and symptoms would point to a pneumothorax. But you've just seen your patient's chest X-ray, so you know his lungs are inflated and there's no air in the pleural space. Consequently, you can shift your suspicions from pneumothorax to another likely culprit such as pulmonary embolism.

Easy to use and understand

The format of *Better X-Ray Interpretation* makes it accessible to a wide range of health care professionals. The first chapter covers the history of radiology, discusses related legal issues, describes imaging techniques, and reviews significant terms used in radiology.

Each of the remaining chapters covers a different body system. After reviewing the anatomy, the chapter describes how key structures normally appear on X-ray films. Next comes a discussion of the imaging techniques used to diagnose the structures and tissues of that body system.

The chapter follows with a description of common diseases and disorders, using a consistent format for each one:
• clinical signs: which symptoms and other clinical findings to expect
• radiographic findings: what various imaging techniques may reveal about the patient's medical condition

• treatment: how the disease or disorder is typically treated
• case study: a chronological account of a patient's hospital stay, correlating his changing medical condition with radiographic findings taken at various stages in his recovery
• guide to patient care: an easy-to-comprehend chart that tells what instructions to give your patient about a given radiologic test and how to care for him before and afterward.

Throughout the book, illustrations depict normal anatomic structures. Most importantly, over 120 photographs of real patients' radiographic images provide an inside-the-body look at common medical conditions. Above each photograph, a clear, concise caption describes exactly what each image shows, with important findings correlated to easy-to-see arrows that appear on the image.

What's more, a glossary at the end of the book defines important radiologic terms. And a comprehensive index makes it easy for readers to find topics of special interest.

Toward better patient care

As health care professionals, we must accept the challenge of radiologic testing as still another tool to help us care for patients more knowledgeably and more efficiently. We're certain that *Better X-Ray Interpretation* will help you meet your growing radiologic responsibilities.

Kathy J. Scheffer, RN
Tacoma General Hospital
Tacoma, Washington

Richard S. Tobin, MD
Tacoma General Hospital
St. Joseph Medical Center
Tacoma, Washington

1 Basic principles of radiology

Radiology entails more than just the familiar, tangible properties of imaging equipment and diagnostic film. This complex branch of modern medicine also encompasses the intangible elements—history, ethics, and standards, for example—that define a discipline's character and form its foundation. An appreciation of these essentials can enhance comprehension of a technical field's clinical components. With that in mind, we begin *Better X-Ray Interpretation* with a look at the development, standards, and nomenclature of radiology.

History of radiology

X-rays were discovered in 1895 by Wilhelm Conrad Roentgen, professor of physics at the University of Würzburg, in Germany. But he wasn't looking for them. He discovered the rays accidentally and named them X-rays—*X* for *unknown.*

Roentgen stumbled on X-rays while experimenting with a cathode ray tube. At the conclusion of an experiment, he noticed that an image had formed on a glass plate while the tube was activated. The discovery was a breakthrough: For the first time, scientists could see structures under the skin. For his discovery, Roentgen won the first Nobel Prize for science in 1901.

Roentgen continued studying the effects of X-rays and developing equipment that produced them, but it was 15 years before X-rays were used in medicine. In the meantime, the French physicist Antoine-Henri Becquerel discovered the radioactivity of uranium, and Marie and Pierre Curie isolated radium, feats for which the three shared the 1903 Nobel Prize for physics. More studies followed, but it wasn't until the 1930s that radiation-safety practices were implemented.

Radiation has been studied extensively since its discovery, and research on its effects and usefulness and its dangers continues.

How X-rays work

X-rays are very short wavelengths of electromagnetic radiation that can penetrate matter. The rays move in waves the way that sound does. X-rays ionize matter or remove an electron from an atom. That's what makes X-rays medically useful—and harmful. X-rays are produced when fast-moving electrons suddenly decelerate after contact with matter, an interaction that produces packets of energy, or photons. The resultant interaction is 99% heat, with X-rays accounting for the remaining 1%.

One of radiation's chief medical uses is to destroy cancer-cell membranes. It can also harm normal tissue, although it affects normal tissue less than it does malignant cells. The body tissues most sensitive to radiation are the lenses of the eyes, those that produce blood, and the gonads.

X-rays interact with matter in several ways, but the two ways that are relevant to diagnostic radiology are the Compton effect (scatter) and the photoelectric effect (absorption). The radiograph (X-ray film) is created when X-rays penetrate the patient and produce different shades from black to white on the film. The different shades are created by the way various body parts absorb the X-ray beam.

X-rays that don't interact with tissue are not absorbed. Instead, they pass through the body unaffected and are responsible for the dark, or high-density, areas on film such as those showing air in the lungs. Gray, or medium-density, areas correspond to body parts with which photoelectric interactions took place or were absorbed, such as tissue or bone.

Scatter radiation, which deflects from the patient and into the radiology suite, has no practical application and is responsible for causing foggy areas on film, making the images diffuse, grayish, and hard to discern. Scatter radiation's relevance to diagnostic radiology is in screening, shielding, and radiation

Basic principles of radiation safety

Time
Duration of exposure

Distance
Exposure decreases with the distance from source according to the inverse-square law. (Doubling distance cuts exposure by 25%.)

Shielding
Protects against scatter radiation; includes aprons, gloves, thyroid shields, leaded or photosensitive glass, and fixed or moveable partitions

safety. Scatter radiation from the patient is nearly as energetic as the primary beam. It accounts for most of radiology personnel's radiation exposure and makes room shielding necessary.

Radiation safety

Radiation protection is important for anyone involved in imaging — patients and personnel.

Patient exposure can be reduced by limiting beam size and exposure with shielding devices (cones, shutters, and gonadal shields), and by covering radiosensitive parts of the patient, such as the eyes and thyroid, with lead glasses and collars.

The three basic principles of radiation safety, also called the cardinal rules of radiation protection, are time, distance, and shielding. (See *Basic principles of radiation safety.*)

• Time is the duration of exposure to ionizing radiation. Halving exposure time cuts the dose in half.

• Distance can provide effective radiation protection. As the distance from the radiation source increases, the dose is reduced according to the inverse-square law. (For instance, when the distance from the X-ray source is doubled, exposure is decreased by one-fourth, or 25%.) Since the primary source of occupational exposure is scatter radiation from the patient, the greatest distance from the patient is the safest. Conventional knowledge has established that a distance of at least 6' (1.8 m) will minimize personnel's radiation exposure.

• Shielding can be used for protection from scatter radiation. Shields protect structures like the thyroid, gonads, and blood-forming tissue. They include lead aprons and gloves, thyroid shields, leaded or photosensitive glass, and permanent or moveable lead-lined partitions.

Monitoring exposure

How much radiation are patients and radiology personnel exposed to? The amount can be tracked and gauged by monitoring devices that measure latent effects of low-level radiation. The devices include film badges, pocket ionization chambers, and thermoluminescent dosimeters.

Film badges are most commonly worn because they're relatively inexpensive and easy to use. They consist of a small strip of film in a light, water-proof packet. Measuring photographic effect on the film, which indicates cumulative exposure in low-exposure areas, gives a good estimate of radiation dose. The badges should not be exposed to heat or water or worn outside work. They should be worn outside of lead aprons at collar level. Workers should have access to monthly film-badge reading reports to gauge their exposure.

Ring badges are available for personnel in nuclear medicine or for those who receive excessive hand exposure because hands are more sensitive to radiation than some other body parts.

Typically, radiation-safety officers, who monitor and report excessive exposure, are assigned to most clinical areas. State, federal, and institutional guidelines help personnel deal with above-average exposures. Reducing exposure may mean taking such steps as rotating clinical assignments to areas of lower exposure for 2 months. The *as low as reasonably accepted* (called ALARA) dose has been set at 150 millirems (mrem) per month.

Pocket ionization chambers are devices that are electrically charged before use. When exposed to ionizing radiation, they lose their charge in proportion to the amount of radiation exposure. Disadvantages of using them include the need for daily readings, their cost, and their decreased sensitivity. They're fragile, but don't wear out easily, and must be re-charged daily.

Thermoluminescent dosimeters use energy-storing crystals to monitor radiation doses. They're worn by workers and are sensitive to low doses of radiation. They can be used for longer periods than pocket ionization chambers. Their high cost, however, is a major deterrent to their widespread use.

How radiation doses are measured

Knowing the level of radiation exposure is important for comparison with national exposure recommendations. The four units of radiation measurement have specific uses but are interrelated. They also have metric, or International System, equivalents. The sievert (Sv) is the international measurement for radiation.

Common units of measurement used in the United States include the following.

• Roentgen (R) is the unit of radiation exposure or intensity.

• The rad is the unit of radiation absorbed dose, which describes the dose received by people or animals.

• The rem, or roentgen equivalent man, quantifies radiation doses for people. The rem takes into account the biological effectiveness of different types of radiation. Its major application is in recording doses from radiation-monitoring devices.

• One Sv is equal to 100 rem.

In diagnostic radiology, the R, rad, and rem measure radiation's biological effects. (See *Common U.S. radiation measurement units*, page 6.)

To minimize occupational injury, the maximum permissible dose (MPD) has been established for various body parts, based on radiosensitivity. (See *Maximum permissible dose*, page 7.)

Radiation protection during pregnancy

Pregnant patients or personnel are a particular concern. When possible, have pregnant women leave the room during radiation exposure.

Common U.S. radiation measurement units

Roentgen (R)
Basic unit of exposure or intensity

Radiation absorbed dose (rad)
Measures human or animal dose

Roentgen equivalent man (rem)
Quantifies human radiation doses; considers biological effectiveness of different radiation types. The major application of rem is for recording doses from radiation-monitoring devices.

Sievert (Sv)
Equal to 100 rem

The 10-day rule of radiation exposure should be followed for women of child-bearing age. The rule states that X-rays in which the primary beam will be directed toward the ovaries should be taken during the first 10 days following the onset of menses to minimize the risk of embryonic radiation exposure.

When an examination can't be postponed until after delivery, the fetus can be protected as much as possible by the use of lead and coning techniques. The radiation dose can be calculated to give the smallest possible exposure. Gestational dosage should not exceed 55 millirem/month. The greatest risk to the fetus is during the first trimester, when organogenesis occurs.

Pregnant personnel should be monitored with two film badges, one worn for maternal scatter at the collar and one worn under the lead apron to measure the fetal dose. When possible, the pregnant worker should not perform fluoroscopy during the first trimester, and participation in the procedure should be limited in the second and third trimesters.

The whole-body dose limit for the 9-month gestational period is 0.5 rem. Maternity lead aprons shield the torso, front, and back. Pregnant personnel should not be assigned to care for radioactive patients, such as those with radium implants. Patients who have had diagnostic or therapeutic irradiation are not considered radioactive.

Maximum permissible dose

Body area	Rem/year	Millisievert (mSv)
Whole body	5 after age 18	50
Hands	75	750
Forearms	30	300
Other organs	15	150

Keep in mind that people are exposed to naturally occurring radiation throughout their lives.

Legal issues

The legal responsibility of any health practitioner is to provide safe care. To this end, the Joint Commission on the Accreditation of Healthcare Organizations and the American College of Radiology (ACR) have established guidelines and standards for safe radiologic care.

Informed consent

Informed consent should be obtained by the radiologist before any complex procedure. The patient should be informed of:
- the nature of the treatment
- any risks, complications, and expected benefits or effects
- alternatives to the procedure and their risks and benefits.

For minors and people with diminished capacity, consent is obtained from a legal guardian or person with power of attorney.

Many institutions use a questionnaire for obtaining informed consent from patients receiving I.V. contrast dye.

Documentation

The patient's medical record or radiology report, or both, must include information from all clinicians who work with the patient to justify diagnosis, course of illness, management, and treatment.

Ownership

Who owns the X-ray film? That's a question patients and doctors have long asked. According to the ACR, "Radiographs are the legal property of the radiologists, physician, or hospital in which they are made."

Films may be lent to the referring doctor but must be returned. X-ray films and reports may be subpoenaed by a court. As with charts, patients can review films if a doctor is available to interpret.

Identification

X-ray films must be properly identified, with the patient's name, X-ray number, date, and institution imprinted on the film. Right and left marks should also be permanently noted on the film.

Record keeping

X-ray films should be filed in the radiology department for 1 year. After that, they should be stored in vaults for a period determined by institutional or state guidelines, or both, if applicable.

Films of minors should be held until the patient is an adult, plus 1 to 3 years, depending on state guidelines. Most mammography films are stored indefinitely for comparison with future films.

Position and projection

Discussion and comprehension of imaging modalities, test results, and therapeutic applications require familiarity with the terminology of radiology. Here's an overview of the words used to describe the positions in which patients are placed for images to be made.

Body position

Body position describes the manner in which a patient is placed for X-rays in relation to surrounding space. It's best for most examinations to get two views of a structure, preferably at right angles to each other, because a dense structure may overlie a less dense structure and obscure it. The size and shape of a body part and its relationship to other structures cannot be appreciated from a single X-ray beam path.

The standard body positions are the frontal and lateral views. Decubitus means lying down. Specific positions are described according to the dependent body surface. The following positions refer to the body surface that's lying on the examination table.

Dorsal recumbent — supine, or lying on back.

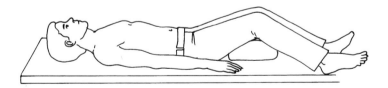

Ventral recumbent — prone, or lying face down.

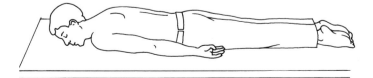

Right lateral recumbent — lying on right side.

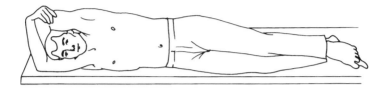

Left lateral recumbent — lying on left side.

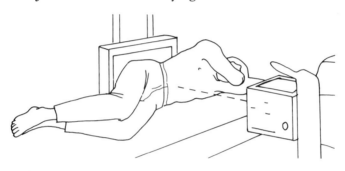

Projection

Projection describes the path of the X-ray beam as it goes from the X-ray tube, through the patient, and onto the film. The view is the representation of an image as seen from the vantage point of the image receptor, or film. Use of the term view is often confused with the term projection. What is commonly referred to as a PA view is actually a PA projection.

Frontal projection

For an anteroposterior (AP) projection, the patient is depicted in the supine or dorsal recumbent body position. The X-ray beam enters the front (anterior) body surface and exits the back (posterior) surface, as shown at the top of the opposite page. This projection is usually done with a portable machine when the patient is unable to travel to the radiology department. The heart may appear enlarged because of its closeness to the X-ray beam.

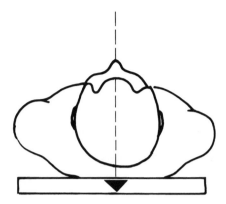

For a posteroanterior (PA) projection, the patient is shown in the upright, or erect, body position. The central ray enters from the rear (posterior) body surface and exits the front (anterior) surface, as shown below. This projection is the standard chest X-ray done in the radiology department.

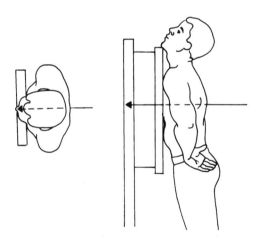

Lateral projection
Lateral projections are always named for the side of the patient that's closer to the film. This projection is helpful in assessing structures posterior to the heart and along the spine

and also the bases of the lung. (See the right lateral projection below.)

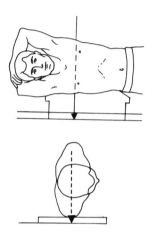

Oblique projection

The term *oblique* refers to a position in which the body part is rotated so that it doesn't produce a frontal (AP or PA) or lateral projection. The oblique projection is helpful in viewing structures at an angle and to move bony structures out of the way of soft-tissue structures. It's also frequently used in angiography to allow vessels to open up or to overcome the problem of overlapping vessels. (See the right PA oblique position below.)

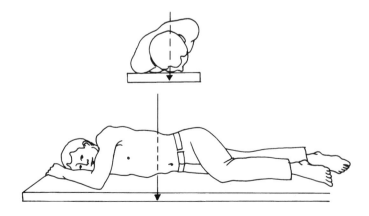

Decubitus (recumbent) projection

Decubitus projection means that the patient is lying down with the central ray parallel to the horizon. In most radiographic decubitus positions, the patient is lying on his side (lateral body surface). Lateral decubitus films help assess for air and fluid levels in the lungs and abdomen. Air will rise to the superior area and fluid will flow dependently to the lowest regions. (See the left lateral decubitus position below.)

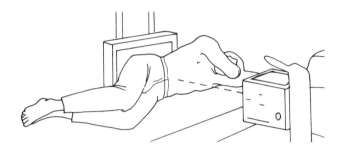

Assessing X-rays

The radiologist assesses and interprets X-ray film. When a nonradiologist assesses a film, it's usually to find an answer to a particular problem or question, such as whether a chest tube or central line is positioned correctly, whether there's fluid in the lungs, or whether the bowel loops are distended.

Comparing any X-ray film with previous films is helpful, particularly when assessing progression of a clinical situation, such as pneumonia or a pneumothorax. The position the film was taken in should be noted. An AP versus a PA projection can change the apparent size of structures because of distance from the X-ray source. For instance, the heart may appear enlarged in an AP projection because it was closer to the X-ray tube (and farther from the film) when exposed.

A decubitus film may be a better projection for assessing fluid levels in the abdomen or chest because the fluid will be in a dependent position. Likewise, the quality and diagnostic usefulness of a portable film taken in a semi-upright position versus a full upright position will be compromised because of fluid collecting in layers posteriorly and because the lungs will not be fully expanded. Often, the health care worker on the patient's unit decides whether the film is made in or out of the radiology department. Although it may be more convenient not to transport the patient, PA and lateral films taken in the radiology department ensure higher image quality and greater diagnostic accuracy.

Differences in film quality, sharpness of detail, patient motion, lightness versus darkness of structures, and patient positioning can all affect the diagnostic usefulness of a radiograph. It's beyond the scope of this book to discuss techniques, exposure factors, and other filming parameters best left to the radiologic technologist and radiologist to determine.

A radiograph should be considered a tool to aid the clinician in confirming a diagnosis or clinical finding. Wheezes or crackles in the lung bases heard on auscultation may be confirmed by the presence of fluid-filled, dense areas seen on a chest X-ray. But often an ordinary radiograph can't give the clinician all the information he needs to make a diagnosis. In that case, he may use another imaging modality to view anatomy or to identify a pathologic process.

Imaging techniques and subspecialties

With technological advancements has come an arsenal of imaging modalities that allow health care professionals to focus on specific body parts in search of particular conditions or diseases. From the proliferation of these technologies have arisen specialities within radiology with which patients can be treated when other treatment methods are inappropriate.

Diagnostic radiology

Diagnostic radiology is where the bread-and-butter films are taken. This branch of radiology includes chest films; abdominal X-rays, like barium enemas and upper GI studies; pharyngograms; genitourinary studies, like excretory urography, cystography, and hystosalpingography; and any plain views of the extremities that are required.

Computed tomography

Computed tomography (CT) scans use ionizing radiation transmitted through the body while an X-ray tube rotates around the patient. Hundreds to thousands of X-ray detectors in the donut-shaped scanner measure the attenuation (or absorption) of X-rays by different tissue. These detectors collect information from each projection, digitize and analyze it by computer, and then reconstruct cross-sectional images, or slices, of the patient. A spiral CT scan, which creates reconstructed, three-dimensional images, can show structures in all projections. Oral and I.V., iodine-based contrast dyes can enhance the image of the area being scanned.

Ultrasonography

Ultrasonography uses sound waves transmitted from a transducer to anatomical structures and converted to electrical impulses on the return echo. These impulses are then converted to an image on the monitor. The brightness of the image corresponds to the strength of the ultrasound echoes. Solid-mass and fluid-filled areas give off different levels of brightness, allowing identification. Ultrasonography is an indispensable diagnostic tool that does not require ionizing radiation and is portable — two attractive qualities.

Magnetic resonance imaging

Magnetic resonance imaging (MRI) is one of the newest diagnostic-imaging techniques. MRI scanners use a magnetic field and radio frequency instead of ionizing radiation to create computer-enhanced images. The images are similar to CT scans in that they are cross-sections, or slices, of the body. Multiple planes, such as the sagittal or coronal, can be reconstructed. With gadolinium contrast agents, a pathologic process is often better appreciated. The main disadvantages of MRI include the length of time patients must remain motionless, the claustrophobic effect of the scanner, and the difficulty of scanning patients with magnetically susceptible devices. Also, MRI remains relatively expensive.

Nuclear medicine

Nuclear medicine is the branch of radiology that uses injected or ingested radioactively tagged compounds. These compounds are preferentially absorbed by their respective target organs. A gamma camera absorbs gamma rays emanating from the patient and transforms the information electronically into an image that can be reproduced on film.

Nuclear medicine has become an important field of imaging because it provides information about organ function and the flow of blood and other body fluids. It's also relatively noninvasive, which makes it a good screening indicator for additional, invasive procedures. For example, a positive ventilation-perfusion ($\dot{V}/\dot{Q}$) scan may indicate the need for pulmonary angiography.

Interventional radiology

With the advent of percutaneous transluminal angioplasty in the 1960s, a whole new field of radiology was born: interventional radiology. Interventional radiology is a subspecialty of radiology that deals not only with diagnosis but also with treatment. Procedures are performed using all available imaging modalities for guidance. Procedures done in a special-procedures suite include angiography; angioplasty; percutaneous gastrostomy-tube placement; biliary-, nephrotomy-, or abscess-catheter placement; embolization of bleeding vessels; infusions of chemotherapeutic drugs directly into the arteries supplying blood flow to the tumors; central venous-line placement; port implantation; and transjugular intrahepatic portocaval systemic shunt placement.

Progress

Radiology has come a long way in the last century, from the accidental discovery of X-rays in a laboratory in Germany to a variety of advanced imaging and treatment techniques in state-of-the-art medical facilities.

With that progress have come new demands on health care workers. And, as the invasiveness and technical demands of procedures have increased, so has the need for highly trained radiologists, nurses, and technologists working as a team.

But those advances and the resulting demands they've placed on health-care workers are increasing the accuracy of diagnoses, enhancing treatment, curing and alleviating disease, and increasing the quality of life of many people worldwide.

Selected references

Ballinger, P.W. *Merrill's Atlas of Radiographic Positions and Radiographic Procedures*, vol. 1, 8th ed. St. Louis: Mosby–Year Book, Inc., 1995.

Dettenmeir, P.A. *A Radiographic Assessment for Nurses*. St. Louis: Mosby–Year Book, Inc., 1995.

Malott, J.C., and Fodor, J., III. *The Art and Science of Medical Radiography*, 7th ed. St. Louis: Mosby–Year Book, Inc., 1993.

Obergfell, A. *Law and Ethics in Diagnostic Imaging*. Philadelphia: W.B. Saunders Co., 1995.

Parelli, R.J. *Medicolegal Issues for Radiographers*. Dubuque, Iowa: Eastwind Publishing, 1994.

Paul, L., and Juhl, J.H. *The Essentials of Roentgen Interpretation*, 3rd ed. New York: Harper & Row Publishers, 1972.

Pizzutiello, R.J., and Cullinan, J.E. *Introduction to Medical Radiographic Imaging*. Rochester, N.Y.: Eastman Kodak, 1995.

2 Respiratory system

The primary function of the respiratory system is to obtain and to help deliver oxygen to the body and to rid the body of carbon dioxide. This vital exchange of gas occurs in the lungs where air is distributed to the alveoli, the tiny air sacs in the lungs. It is in the alveoli that blood takes on oxygen and gives off carbon dioxide. The respiratory system is usually divided into two tracts: the upper respiratory tract and the lower respiratory tract.

Anatomy

On an adult's chest X-ray, the heart, lungs, bony thorax, diaphragm, clavicles, and scapulae are outlined, and the chest wall's soft tissue is also seen. The thorax is divided by the mediastinum into two compartments, each containing an air-filled lung, both of which are relatively radiolucent compared with the mediastinum, chest wall, and upper abdominal viscera. Most of the trachea is also visible.

A basic knowledge of the location and functions of the lower respiratory tract is needed to understand a pathologic process and to interpret radiographic findings. The next few pages summarize the appearance of soft tissue, bony thorax, pleura, lungs, trachea, mediastinum, and diaphragm and describe these structures' radiographic interpretation.

Soft tissue
Soft tissue surrounding the bony thorax may produce dense areas that overlie lung tissue and simulate disease findings. Skin folds can produce linear shadows, and breast-tissue shadows show up on film. Lateral soft tissue should be of the same thickness and density. A matted appearance is usually abnormal and suggests subcutaneous emphysema brought on by a pneumothorax.

Bony thorax

The bony thorax includes the thoracic vertebrae, ribs, sternum, and costal cartilage that secures the ribs to the sternum. The clavicles (anterior) and scapulae (posterior) make up the shoulder girdle.

On normal inspiratory chest film, eight to nine anterior ribs should overlie lung tissue. When fewer than eight ribs overlie lung tissue, suspect small lung volume or poor inspiratory effort. Inspect the clavicles for fractures. The medial head should lie directly over the vertebral column.

The scapulae are also assessed for injury and position. On an anteroposterior (AP) film, the scapulae may be mistaken for a pneumothorax. Avoid this mistake by looking for lung markings past the scapula line. The posteroanterior (PA) projection is preferred because the scapulae separate as the shoulders roll forward and more of the lung field is visible. (See "Position and projection," page 9.)

Pleura

The pleura is divided into two sections, visceral and parietal. The visceral pleura covers each lobe of the chest; the parietal pleura covers the diaphragm and lines the thorax. The pleura isn't usually seen in the normal X-ray, but it may appear as a thin outer wall of the lung when pneumothorax is present. The two pleurae are separated by a potential space that holds the 25 ml of surfactant needed to prevent friction as the lungs expand and contract.

Lungs

The lungs occupy all of the thoracic cavity, except for the mediastinum. Each lung is suspended by vascular and bronchial attachments called roots. The highest portion of each lung is the apex. The concave lower surface that rests on the diaphragm is the base. The hilus is the medial (mediastinal) indentation through which blood vessels enter and leave the lung. The primary bronchi enter through the hilus and then separate into smaller branches.

The left lung is smaller, with a cardiac notch to accommodate the heart, and is divided into two lobes by the oblique fissure, which is best seen on the lateral chest film.

The right lung has three lobes separated by the horizontal fissure and the oblique fissure.

The lungs are air-filled and should appear radiolucent, or black, when compared with the fluid-filled heart or with the dense bones.

Three different lung markings are associated with various pathologic processes represented by increased radiopacity (whiteness). They are alveolar, interstitial, or vascular patterns noted in the lung fields. Their significance and appearance will be explained later in this chapter.

Trachea
The trachea, or windpipe, is an air-filled elastic tube that enters the mediastinum at the T5 level and bifurcates at the carina into the right and left primary bronchi. Because it's air-filled, the trachea will appear radiolucent on film and should be midline in normal position.

Mediastinum
The central area of the thoracic cavity is called the mediastinum. It houses the heart, great vessels, bronchi, esophagus, and thymus. The sternum is anterior to the mediastinum and protects the vital organs. The heart is normally 12 cm long, 9 cm wide, and 6 cm deep. The heart extends more to the left when ventricular hypertrophy or cardiomegaly is present.

Diaphragm
The diaphragm makes up the base of the thoracic cavity. It's a broad domelike muscle when relaxed (expiration), and when contracted (inspiration), it flattens and moves upward. The diaphragm is the principal muscle of inspiration. The diaphragm's lateral borders make up the sharp, pointed costophrenic angles, whereas the medial cardiophrenic angle is less sharp. When either or both the costophrenic or cardiophrenic angles are blunted, suspect pleural effusion.

The right diaphragm is 1 to 2 cm higher than the left. On deep inspiration, the diaphragm moves 3 to 5 cm.

Imaging techniques

The full spectrum of imaging techniques, from plain X-rays to the ventilation-perfusion scan of nuclear medicine, makes it possible for health care professionals to see the structures of the respiratory system.

X-ray

X-rays are the most common diagnostic tool used to make images of the chest. They're used to screen, diagnose, and evaluate changing patient status. Standard chest X-ray projections are the PA and lateral. For a portable chest X-ray, the AP projection is usually used.

Position should be noted on the film and considered when assessing an X-ray. On an AP view, the heart may appear enlarged or magnified because it's closer to the X-ray tube. Other projections, such as oblique or lordotic, may help in accessing a particular structure or to note whether a chest lesion is anterior or posterior. (See *Normal posteroanterior chest X-ray*, page 22.)

Ultrasonography

Ultrasonography produces images by converting sound waves returning from the body in echoes into electrical impulses. These echoes are received by a transducer, which translates the electrical impulses into images that then appear on a monitor. Ultrasonography is used primarily on the chest to view fluid collections and to aid in thoracentesis. Its portability is one of its best features.

Computed tomography

Computed tomography (CT) scanning uses ionizing radiation and computer reconstruction to show anatomic structures in cross-sections, or slices. CT scanning is an excellent way to

Normal posteroanterior chest X-ray

This X-ray shows certain normal, soft, and bony structures in the chest and upper abdomen.

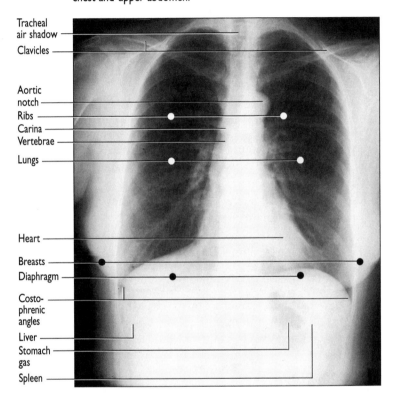

Tracheal air shadow
Clavicles
Aortic notch
Ribs
Carina
Vertebrae
Lungs
Heart
Breasts
Diaphragm
Costo- phrenic angles
Liver
Stomach gas
Spleen

visualize small lesions or fluid collections and to locate their exact position. It helps radiologists perform lung biopsy and fluid drainage and assess the mediastinum and hilar regions. (See *CT scans of the chest.*)

Angiography

A pulmonary angiogram detects pulmonary emboli or infarction when a nuclear-medicine scan is inconclusive. Angiography is more invasive and more risky, but is considered the

CT scans of the chest

These CT scans were taken at the level of the tracheal bifurcation. Figure A shows hilar and mediastinal anatomy. Note ascending aorta **AA**, descending aorta **DA**, pulmonary artery **PA**, superior vena cava **S**, and esophagus E. Ribs, vertebra, and scapula are shown. Figure B shows lung detail. Note carina→, lung →, and pulmonary vascularity →. This patient has undergone coronary artery bypass graft, and sternal wires and surgical clips are seen.

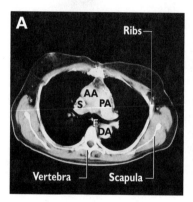

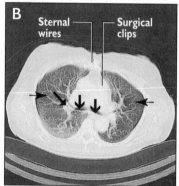

definitive examination for diagnosing pulmonary emboli. A contrast dye is injected via a pulmonary-artery catheter, with sequential films taken during injection.

Ventilation-perfusion scan

In a ventilation-perfusion ($\dot{V}/\dot{Q}$) scan, , which is part of nuclear medicine, a small amount of a radioisotope is injected I.V. to assess perfusion (blood flow), and a second radiopharmaceutical agent is inhaled through a nebulizer to assess ventilation (gas exchange) in a lung segment. Scanning locates areas of mismatched ventilation and blood perfusion. A mismatch may indicate a pulmonary embolism. (See *Guide to patient care*, page 66, for guidelines on preparing patients for various types of imaging.)

Pathophysiology

A host of conditions can compromise the integrity and functions of the respiratory system. Many of these conditions, whether caused by disease or trauma, are life-threatening. This chapter will help health care professionals recognize disease and other processes at work in the respiratory system, what they look like in X-rays or other diagnostic radiologic images, and what treatment may be administered.

Atelectasis

Atelectasis, or collapse of lung tissue, is always a secondary process and a sign of disease, not a disease itself. The two categories of atelectasis are compression and absorption.

Compression atelectasis is caused by external pressure — from a tumor, fluid, or air in the pleural space. Increased abdominal pressure on a portion of the lung can cause alveolar collapse.

Absorption atelectasis results from removal of air from obstructed or hypoventilated alveoli. This can occur when a bronchus is obstructed or after concentrated oxygen or anesthetics are inhaled.

Atelectasis tends to occur postoperatively from oxygen and anesthetics used in surgery. Increased pain, shallow breathing, reluctance to move, and viscous secretions that pool dependently can cause atelectasis.

⇔ Clinical signs

Signs and symptoms of atelectasis are similar to those of pulmonary infections and include dyspnea, cough, fever, and leukocytosis.

⇔ Radiographic findings

Classic X-ray findings in a patient with atelectasis include the following:
  • elevation of the diaphragm

• a shift of the mediastinum to the side of involvement
• narrowing of the rib interspaces
• trachea possibly deviated toward the affected side
• lack of air in the affected portion of the lung causing an
area of increased density, which is uniform and may appear
linear (in discoid atelectasis) or may involve a segment or lobe
or an entire lung. (See *Small cell lung cancer,* page 26, and
Effects of small cell lung cancer, page 27.)

➪ Treatment

Prevention and treatment include deep-breathing exercises,
incentive spirometry, frequent position changes, and early
ambulation.

Infiltrates

Infiltrates are fluid-filled air spaces that are radiopaque on
film. They often follow atelectasis and may be acute (pneumonia) or chronic (tuberculosis, cystic fibrosis, or bronchiectasis).

➪ Clinical signs

Patients with acute infiltrates exhibit signs and symptoms of
pneumonia, such as shortness of breath, fever, chills, productive cough, and diaphoresis.

Breath sounds may be diminished. Crackles and wheezes
may be present. Patients with chronic infiltrates may be
asymptomatic or may exhibit some of the same manifestations
as with acute infiltrates.

➪ Radiographic findings

X-ray findings of infiltrates follow:
• Fluid-filled air spaces will appear white on film. When
two fluid-filled areas are next to each other, they blur together,
obliterating the borders between the air spaces.
• Infiltrates next to the heart will blur the cardiac borders.
This is called the *silhouette sign,* and can also refer to the loss

Small cell lung cancer

This posteroanterior chest X-ray is from a 54-year-old man with small cell lung cancer and left upper lobe atelectasis. Note left upper lobe density ⇒ indicative of atelectasis, left hilar mass ➤, with elevation of the left hilum and tenting of the left hemidiaphragm ➜ caused by the atelectasis.

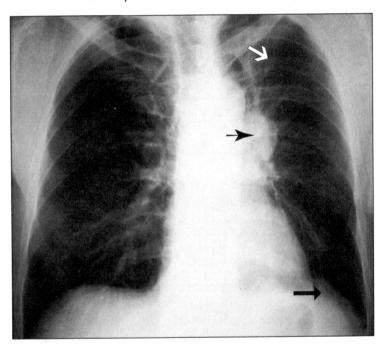

of the diaphragmatic border. (See *Pulmonary infiltrates*, page 28, *Lobar pneumonia*, page 29, and *Lateral chest X-ray of pulmonary infiltrate*, page 30.)

• In severe cases, the trachea may be deviated toward the unaffected side.

⇔ Treatment

Antibiotics may be used if accumulated fluid is infected. Deep breathing, along with coughing and chest physiotherapy, may

Effects of small cell lung cancer

This lateral chest X-ray shows atelectatic changes. Note anterior displacement of the major fissure ⇒ and elevated left hemidiaphragm ⇢. The spine is curved ⟹ because the patient also has ankylosing spondylitis.

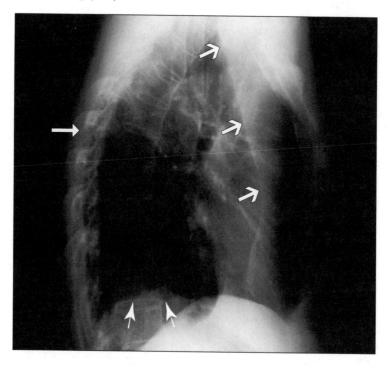

help expel mucus. A chest X-ray can help determine which lobe is involved and how to position the patient for postural drainage.

Pulmonary edema

Pulmonary edema is excessive water in the lung. It most commonly results from left-sided heart failure. It may also be caused by adult respiratory distress syndrome (ARDS). Predisposing factors include barbiturate and opiate poisoning, pneumonia, inhalation of irritating gases, and mitral stenosis.

Pulmonary infiltrates

This anteroposterior chest X-ray shows a right upper lobe infiltrate, which frequently accompanies pneumonia ⇒, and a less conspicuous left lower infiltrate ➤. Note also endotracheal tube ⇒ and pulmonary artery catheter ▷.

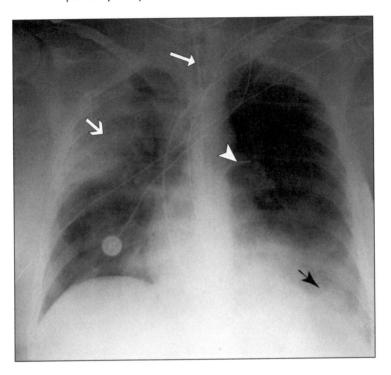

⇨ Clinical signs

Signs of pulmonary edema include dyspnea, hypoxemia, and pink, frothy sputum.

Pulmonary edema may be acute or chronic, depending on the underlying cause. Further classification is based on the area of fluid accumulation: interstitial or alveolar.

Lobar pneumonia

This chest X-ray of a 79-year-old woman shows classic findings of lobar pneumonia involving the left lower lobe ⇒. The classic signs are the silhouette sign, in which the left hemidiaphragm and heart shadow borders can't be seen, mild atelecstasis (note smaller left lung), and depressed left hilum with mediastinal shift to the left ➤.

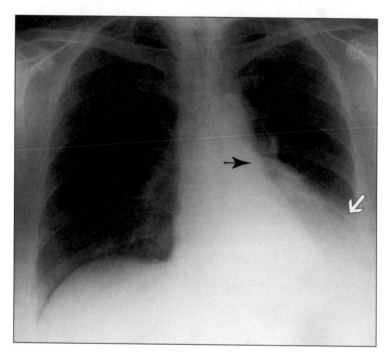

Radiographic findings

The radiographic manifestations of interstitial and alveolar edema vary.

Interstitial edema is usually less severe than alveolar edema. Five classic X-ray findings in interstitial edema are:
- appearance of septal lines
- perivascular blurring where margins of vessels are indistinct
- hilar haze, which refers to loss of definition of large cen-

Lateral chest X-ray of pulmonary infiltrate

Note the sharp upper border of the infiltrate defined by the major fissure ➡. The right hemidiaphragm is clearly seen ➤, but the left is obscured by the infiltrates.

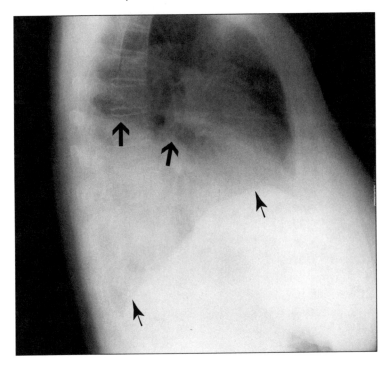

tral pulmonary vessels with slight increase in density
• diffuse reticular patttern that's visible when fluid widens interstitial structures throughout the lungs (see *Interstitial pulmonary edema*, page 32)
• enlarged heart, dilated vessels, and pleural effusion when secondary to congestive heart failure.

Alveolar edema may result from interstitial edema and usually indicates more severe edema.

Classic X-ray findings are:
• bilateral, dense areas extending in a fan-shaped manner from the hilum

• relatively clear peripheral lung fields

• pulmonary edema caused by cardiac disease usually showing an enlarged heart, pulmonary congestion, and pleural effusion

• pulmonary edema caused by uremia producing a classic, fluffy, dense area in the lungs without cardiac enlargement or pulmonary congestion. (See *Alveolar pulmonary edema*, page 33.)

Treatment

Treatment of pulmonary edema depends on its cause. If the cause is cardiac, then diuretics, vasodilators, and medications that increase myocardial contractility are prescribed.

Pulmonary edema associated with ARDS requires interventions that are designed to decrease capillary leakage. For instance, the doctor may order such treatments as colloidal agents, pulmonary end-expiratory pressure (PEEP) ventilation, and supplemental oxygen.

Tracheal deviation

The trachea is normally in a midline position. When it shifts left or right, it's said to have deviated. Deviation may occur from atelectasis (a shift to the collapsed side) or from pressure exerted by fluid, pneumothorax, enlarged lymph nodes, or a mass.

Clinical signs

Clinical signs depend on the cause of the deviation. (See "Atelectasis," page 24, "Pneumothorax," page 38, "Pleural effusion," page 41, and "Lung cancer," page 50.)

Radiographic findings

On chest X-rays, the trachea is shifted to one side. The causes of the deviation must be identified. For instance, imaging studies may yield findings of conditions, such as pneumothorax, hemothorax, tumor, atelectasis, enlarged lymph nodes, or

Interstitial pulmonary edema

This posteroanterior chest X-ray reveals interstitial pulmonary edema. Note septal lines ➔ and diffuse, reticular pattern ➤.

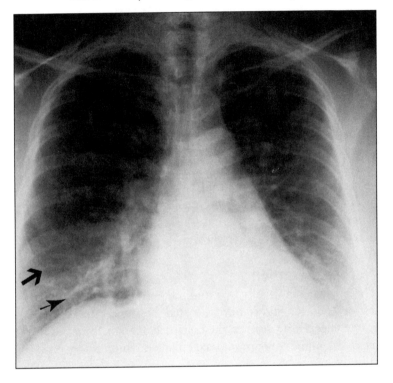

severe pulmonary edema. Separate studies may be required to provide details on the underlying cause of the deviation.

⤳ Treatment

Tracheal deviation is caused by an underlying condition that acts on the trachea to push it away from the midline position. Treating the cause of tracheal deviation will help to relieve it and cause a shift back to midline.

Alveolar pulmonary edema

This anteroposterior chest X-ray shows pulmonary edema. Note the diffuse, bilateral, fluffy infiltrates ➜, which represent the predominantly alveolar edema.

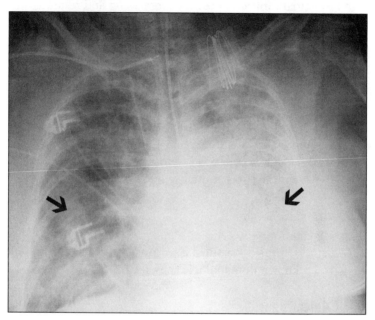

Adult respiratory distress syndrome

ARDS is characterized by diffuse alveolocapillary injury, which leads to acute pulmonary congestion and edema without cardiac involvement. Causes may be major trauma; septicemia; a near drowning incident; inhalation of toxic fumes; severe burns; central nervous system injuries; or other severe, and often multisystemic, processes.

➪ Clinical signs

Signs include rapid, shallow breathing; respiratory alkalosis; marked dyspnea; decreased lung compliance; and hypoxemia unresponsive to oxygen treatment.

⇨ Radiographic findings

Serial chest X-ray findings include:
• diffuse infiltration without evidence of cardiac disease
• interstitial infiltrates possibly progressing and resulting in alveolar infiltrates
• usually, the absence of effusions and cardiac enlargement.

⇨ Treatment

Treatment of ARDS depends on early detection by chest X-rays, arterial blood gas (ABG) analysis, and physical examination. Fluid management, oxygen administration, PEEP ventilation, and cardiovascular and steroid drugs are used to treat ARDS, which has a 50% mortality rate despite treatment.

Asthma

This is a condition involving episodic periods of bronchospasm. Asthma is classified as extrinsic, allergic, or intrinsic with no known immunologic cause.

⇨ Clinical signs

Clinical signs of asthma include dyspnea with marked respiratory effort, inspiratory and expiratory wheezing, nonproductive cough, prolonged expiration, tachycardia, and tachypnea.

⇨ Radiographic findings

Chest X-rays may show:
• hyperenflation with areas of focal atelectasis
• opacifications if the bronchial lining thickens. (See *Pulmonary changes with asthma,* page 36.)

⇨ Treatment

The causative agent, if known, needs to be removed. Bronchodilators, atropine-like medications, theophylline, and supportive oxygen therapy to maintain a partial pressure of arterial oxygen (PaO_2) above 50 mm Hg, and corticosteroids to decrease inflammation are used.

Chronic obstructive pulmonary disease

Chronic obstructive pulmonary disease (COPD) is characterized by difficult expiration. The primary cause is cigarette smoking. Many experts differentiate COPD caused by chronic bronchitis from that caused by emphysema.

Chronic bronchitis

This inflammation of the bronchi is caused by irritants such as cigarette smoke, or infection. It can be acute or chronic and is characterized by increased mucus-productive cough, mucosal swelling, and impaired ciliary function.

➯ Clinical signs

Signs of chronic bronchitis include prolonged expiration, productive cough, chronic hypoventilation, polycythemia, and cyanosis. The patient may have a history of smoking.

Diagnosis is based on physical examination, chest X-ray, pulmonary function tests, and ABG levels.

➯ Radiographic findings

Chest X-rays in chronic bronchitis may show:
- hyperinflation of the lungs
- increased bronchovascular markings.

➯ Treatment

The best treatment is prevention by cessation of smoking. Bronchodilators, expectorants, and chest physiotherapy are commonly used. Low-level oxygen therapy may be used to avoid increasing PaO_2 levels above 60 mm Hg.

Pulmonary changes with asthma

In this posteroanterior chest X-ray of a young woman with asthma, note the hyperinflated lungs ➜, small heart ➞, and depressed diaphragm ➡.

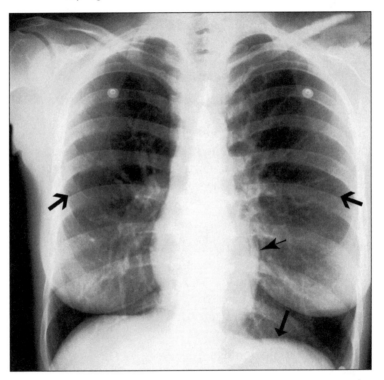

Emphysema

Emphysema is an abnormal, permanent enlargement of the gas-exchange airways accompanied by destruction of alveolar walls. Expiration becomes difficult because of the loss of elastic recoil and partial airway collapse.

↪ Clinical signs

The signs of emphysema include prolonged expiration, productive cough, barrel chest, chronic hypoventilation, and

Pulmonary changes with chronic obstructive pulmonary disease

In this posteroanterior chest X-ray of a patient with chronic obstructive pulmonary disease, Note the large bullae characteristic of emphysema ➜, shown as lucency in the left upper chest.

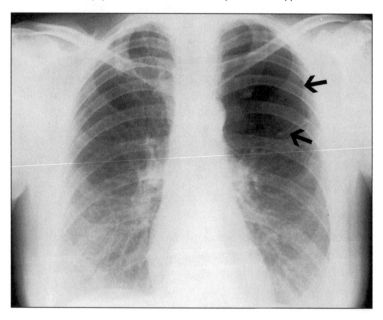

polycythemia (late in the course of the illness). The patient may have a history of smoking.

⟳ Radiographic findings

The most definitive evidence of emphysema can be seen on a chest X-ray. Findings include:
- elongated cardiac silhouette
- highly visible aortic arch
- increased bilateral low-lung field radiolucency
- flattened diaphragms (usually)
- bullae. (See *Pulmonary changes with chronic obstructive pulmonary disease.)*

⟜ Treatment

Cessation of smoking or ending inhalation of other respiratory irritants, preferably both, is essential in the treatment of COPD. Low-flow oxygen therapy is used to treat hypoxia. Breathing exercises, such as pursed-lip breathing, are taught to help compensate for incomplete expiration of air and to slow exhalation and prevent alveolar collapse. Hydration should be increased to 3 L per day. Bronchodilators and steroids may ease respiratory effort. In selected patients, chest physiotherapy is performed to mobilize secretions. Antibiotics are given to treat any respiratory infections. Flu vaccine is given to prevent influenza and Pneumovax is given to prevent pneumococcal pneumonia. Teach the patient and family about appropriate rest so the maneuvers can be done properly to achieve maximum benefit.

Pneumothorax

Pneumothorax is the presence of air or gas in the pleural potential space from a ruptured visceral pleura, or air trapped between the parietal pleura and chest wall. The negative pressure of the pleural space is destroyed, which causes the lung to collapse toward the hilus. There are two types of pneumothorax: open and tension.

Open, or communicating, pneumothorax occurs when air pressure in the pleural space equals barometric pressure, such as when there is an open chest wound into the pleural space.

Tension pneumothorax, in which pleural-space air can't escape through the rupture, is a life-threatening emergency. This type of pneumothorax, which occurs unexpectedly—most often in healthy young men—is caused by ruptured blebs on the visceral pleura, usually in the apices of the lung. Air pressure in the pleural space pushes against the recoiled lung, causing compression atelectasis. Air also presses against the mediastinum, compressing and displacing the heart and great vessels.

Pneumothorax

In this posteroanterior chest X-ray, a small pneumothorax is present in the left lung ➔. Note placement of chest tube ➤, which allows for lung reinflation.

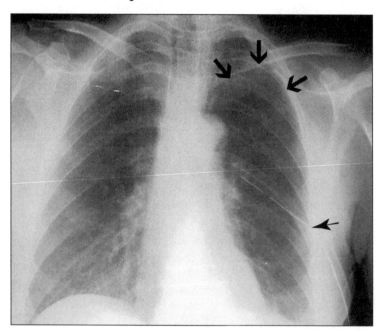

⟳ Clinical signs

For pneumothorax, signs include sudden, sharp, pleuritic pain; asymmetric chest wall movement; shortness of breath and cyanosis; anxiety; tachypnea; and weak, rapid pulse. Tension pneumothorax causes more severe respiratory symptoms.

⟳ Radiographic findings

Chest X-ray findings in pneumothorax include the following.
  • The visceral pleural line usually is fairly easy to see.
  • If there's a large pneumomediastinal shift to the affected side, lung compression and diaphragm depression occur.

Pneumothorax with subcutaneous emphysema

In this posteroanterior chest X-ray of a patient with a pneumothorax, the chest tube ⇒ has migrated outside of the pleural space. As a result, the patient has a larger pneumothorax →▷ than was present originally. The patient has also developed subcutaneous and mediastinal emphysema ⟹.

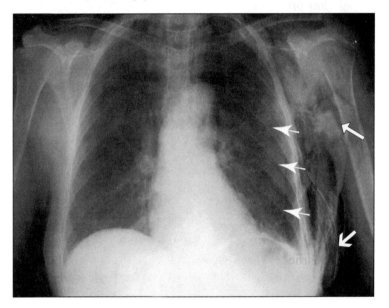

• The trachea may be deviated toward the unaffected side.

• A chest X-ray taken during expiration helps detect a small pneumothorax because lung tissue is denser than air, and so lung volume will decrease during expiration, but the pneumothorax space will not change. Progress films are used to follow its course. (See *Pneumothorax*, page 39, and *Pneumothorax with subcutaneous emphysema*.)

⇨ Treatment

Treatment of both types of pneumothorax requires immediate placement of a chest tube connected to water-seal drainage and suction until the damaged pleura is healed.

Pleural effusion

This is a collection of fluid in the pleural space. Pleural effusion is not a disease in itself, but a sign of disease. The fluid source is usually a leak from small veins or lymphatic vessels under the pleura, or it may come from an abscess or a lesion draining into the pleural space. The fluid is classified as transudate (low protein content) or exudate (high protein content).

➡ Clinical signs

Clinical signs depend on the amount of fluid in the pleural space. A large effusion can cause dyspnea. Compression atelectasis with impaired ventilation and mediastinal shift can occur. Pleural pain is present if the pleura is inflamed.

➡ Radiographic findings

In plain chest X-rays, the fluid level in the pleural space must be above 250 ml to be evident. Other findings include the following.

• The earliest sign of fluid on an upright chest X-ray is obliteration of the sharp angle produced by the normal costophrenic sulcus.

• Increasing fluid will obscure the diaphragm and basal lung fields.

• The superior border of the fluid is often concave and blurred.

• As the effusion progresses, there is compression of the lung and depression of the diaphragm.

• There may also be a mediastinal shift to the opposite side. (See *Pleural effusion,* page 42, and *Pleural effusion with fluid in fissures,* page 43.)

➡ Treatment

Small effusions — usually taken care of by the body itself and drained internally by the lymphatic system — don't require treatment. Thoracentesis is performed if pulmonary function

Pleural effusion

This is a posteroanterior chest X-ray of a 58-year-old man with a history of congestive heart failure. The patient has right-side pleural fluid blunting the right costophrenic angle due to the pleural fluid. Note concavity of the upper border of the pleural fluid ➔.

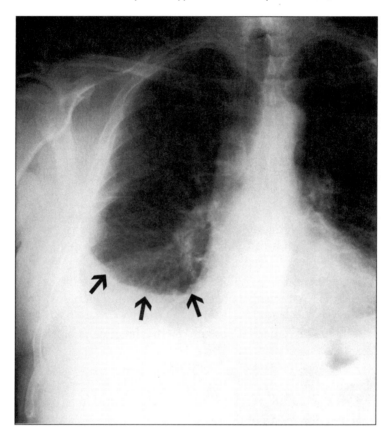

is impaired. Antibiotics are used if the fluid is infected, and steroids may be given to decrease inflammation. Diuretics may help to resolve the problem if the cause of the effusion is cardiac. The course of treatment for most large effusions is determined by tapping the fluid by thoracentesis and analyzing it for infection or other clues to its nature.

Pleural effusion with fluid in fissures

This lateral chest X-ray of the patient whose X-ray appears on the opposite page shows pleural fluid in the lung fissures ➔, which is demonstrated more clearly on a lateral X-ray. Fissures are the spaces between lobes of the lungs that have been widened by fluid.

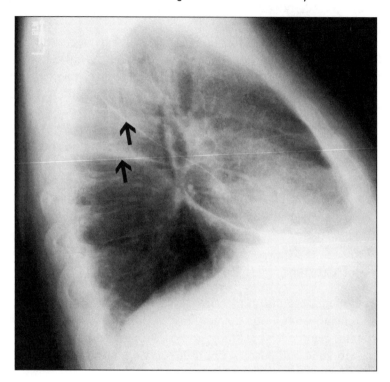

Pneumonia

Pneumonia is an acute infection of the lung caused primarily by bacteria or viruses. Pathogenic microorganisms may reach the lungs by inhalation, aspiration, or hematogenous routes.

➔ Clinical signs

Most cases of pneumonia are preceded by upper respiratory infection, which is frequently viral. It progresses to fever, chills, productive or dry cough, malaise, pleural pain and, sometimes, dyspnea and hemoptysis.

➥ Radiographic findings

Plain chest X-ray findings of pneumonia include the following.

• Lobar, or bacterial, pneumonia causes a mass of consolidated fluid in one or more lobes. A lateral chest X-ray may define the degree of segmental involvement. The silhouette sign with obliteration of cardiac or diaphragmatic borders adjacent to the pneumonia is common.

• Lobular, or bronchopneumonia, is a patchy, irregular distribution involving all structures (bronchi, bronchioles, and alveoli) usually localized in one or more lobes around the bronchi.

• Interstitial, or viral, pneumonia appears more diffuse and is usually less densely consolidated. It may have a more reticular pattern.

➥ Treatment

Treatment depends on identifying the appropriate organism and includes antibiotic therapy, increased fluids, frequent coughing and deep breathing, and chest physiotherapy, including vibration and postural drainage every 4 hours. Oxygen is administered to improve oxygenation.

Tuberculosis

TB is caused by *Mycobacterium tuberculosis,* an acid-fast bacillus that usually affects the lungs but may affect other body systems. The bacillus is transported through air-borne droplets inhaled into the bronchi. It may then cause an acute pneumonitis or primary active TB. More commonly, the bacillus is isolated and walled off by the immune system. It can lie dormant in the host for life, but can be reactivated whenever the immune system is impaired or compromised. Then, the condition is referred to as reinfectious, or secondary, TB.

⮑ Clinical signs

Initially, infected patients are usually asymptomatic. In other patients, symptoms progress gradually until the disease is advanced. Fatigue, weight loss, lethargy, anorexia, and low-grade fever are common manifestations. A cough that produces purulent sputum develops slowly and gradually worsens. Night sweats and general anxiety are usually present.

⮑ Radiographic findings

• On plain chest X-rays, primary TB appears as a small infiltrate with low density, usually limited to a subsegment of the lung.

• Serial chest films obtained over 6 months to 1 year show slow resolution of the infiltrate, which may resolve completely. Often, a small calcified nodule will be noted in X-rays later, with calcification present in the hilar nodes.

• In secondary TB, reinfection most commonly occurs in the upper lobes of the lungs. Lymph-node involvement is less common here than in primary TB.

• On a plain chest X-ray, secondary TB appears as an area of mottled density that may vary greatly in size.

As the disease advances, chest X-rays may show calcification, fibrosis, and tuberculoma with calcium in them. (See *Secondary TB,* page 47.)

⮑ Treatment

Treatment begins following positive skin test, sputum culture, and a chest X-ray. It consists of a 9- to 18-month course of antibiotics. Two or more antibiotics (such as isoniazid, rifampin, ethambutol, and streptomycin) are used to prevent drug-resistant strains of TB from emerging.

Rib fractures

Fractures of the ribs are the most common type of chest trauma. The main complication associated with rib fractures is damage to the pleura or lungs. Bleeding into the pleural space and pneumothorax are potentially serious accompanying problems.

⇨ Clinical signs

Pain at the site of injury, especially on inspiration, is the primary manifestation. Shallow breathing and splinting of the affected side are often observed. Atelectasis may occur from decreased ventilation and lung expansion.

⇨ Radiographic findings

Complete rib fractures with displacement of fragments are fairly easy to discern on a PA chest X-ray, but special rib film techniques and oblique angles may be needed to recognize hairline, incomplete, or buckling fractures. Often, the presence of cloudy periosteal callus several weeks after the injury will indicate healing fractures that were not seen before. (See *Rib fractures*, page 48.)

⇨ Treatment

Intercostal-nerve blocks of the fracture site and at the two ribs above and below the site are performed to decrease pain. The main goal of treatment is to reduce pain and to promote adequate respiration and lung expansion. Judicious use of narcotics is required because they depress respirations. Chest tubes may be required to treat hemothorax or pneumothorax. (See "Case study: Chest trauma," page 63.)

Flail chest

Flail chest is one of the most serious complications of rib fractures. It occurs when a portion of the chest wall caves in as the result of several severe rib fractures. The chest wall then can't provide the necessary support of the lungs for adequate ventilation. During inspiration, the chest moves inward, causing mediastinal shift away from the injury. The reverse occurs during expiration.

Secondary TB

This posteroanterior chest X-ray of a 47-year-old man with reactivated (secondary) tuberculosis shows a mass-like infiltrate with cavitation ➜ and some associated calcification. Left lower lobe infiltrate is present secondary to spillage of infected material into the bronchus ⇢.

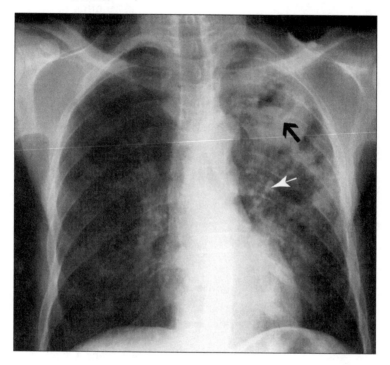

➪ Clinical signs

Look for these signs of flail chest: pain, dyspnea, unequal chest expansion, hypoventilation, and hypoxemia. As the patient worsens, look for cyanosis, tachycardia, and tachypnea.

➪ Radiographic findings

Look for the following chest X-ray findings indicating flail chest:

Rib fractures

This anteroposterior chest X-ray of a trauma patient after a motor vehicle accident shows left fifth ➜ and sixth ➤ lateral rib fractures. Note separation at fracture sites due to displacement and associated left clavicle ➜ and left scapula fractures ▶.

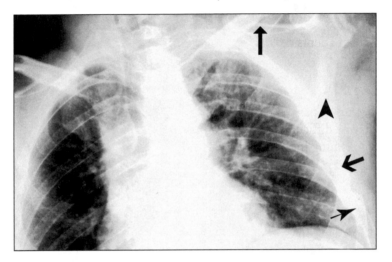

  • rib fractures, which are usually easy to see because several severe fractures occur
    • mediastinal shifting during inspirations
    • atelectasis
    • pneumothorax.
Hemothorax is also usually present. (Associated abdominal and cardiac or vascular injuries are common.)

↪ Treatment

Once the diagnosis is made by chest X-ray, adequate ventilation is the main concern. Oxygen therapy and chest reexpansion are critical. Intubation and mechanical ventilation are often needed initially to aid lung expansion and to help the lung parenchyma to heal.

Ruptured or perforated diaphragm

Blunt or sharp penetrating trauma to the diaphragm may cause a tear or perforation. Depending on the site, abdominal contents herniate through the perforation.

➯ Clinical signs

Most patients complain of chest pain in the shoulders or of pain in the abdomen. Dyspnea, tachypnea, and shallow breathing are present. Diaphragmatic or respiratory movement is decreased. Bowel sounds may be heard high in the chest if the bowel has perforated it. Passing a nasogastric (NG) tube may be difficult. A ruptured diaphragm is often a life-threatening injury.

➯ Radiographic findings

It may be difficult to detect a ruptured or perforated diaphragm on chest X-rays. Considering associated findings and the whole clinical picture will aid in diagnosing the tear. Serial films may be needed to show differences in the hemidiaphragm heights and presence of bowel or stomach in the thoracic cavity.

If the pleura was damaged at the time of injury, a pneumothorax may be present. If the injury to the diaphragm is not found initially, inflammation eventually occurs and will cause:
- basilar congestion
- pleural inflammation with fluid buildup
- noticeable elevation of the diaphragm.

➯ Treatment

Surgical repair is required. Patients are often severely ill, and most will have associated injuries to abdominal organs. An NG tube is placed carefully to keep the stomach evacuated. I.V. fluids, antibiotics, and supportive care are provided until surgery can be performed.

Lung cancer

Lung cancer is the leading cause of cancer deaths in the United States. It's most common in adults older than age 50 with a history of smoking. Cigarette smoking causes a change in the bronchial epithelium that usually returns to normal when smoking is discontinued. Another risk factor is inhalation of carcinogens. Asbestos, nickel, iron, uranium, arsenic, air pollution, and polycyclic aromatic hydrocarbons are carcinogenic.

Cancers originate in the bronchial epithelium more than 90% of the time. They grow slowly and can take up to 10 years to reach an X-ray-detectable 1 cm. Primary lung cancers are categorized by their histological types. Metastasis occurs by direct extension into the lung and via the blood and lymph systems. Liver, brain, bones, lymph nodes, and adrenal glands are common metastatic sites.

Clinical signs

Most signs occur late in the disease process. Persistent pneumonitis caused by obstructed bronchi may be an early sign causing fever, chills, and cough. A productive, persistent cough is a significant early symptom. Later symptoms include anorexia, fatigue, weight loss, nausea, and vomiting.

Diagnostic tests include chest X-ray, CT scan, and nuclear studies. Bronchoscopy, sputum sampling, and needle biopsy aid diagnosis.

Radiographic findings

Initial X-ray findings may include:
- atelectasis, which may be segmental or lobar
- unilateral hilar enlargement
- obstructive emphysema
- mediastinal mass
- apical mass
- segmental density that doesn't clear
- a tumor that may appear as an opaque (often round), dense area

Lung cancer

This is a chest X-ray of a 67-year-old woman with bronchogenic lung cancer. Note the large mass → with cavitation at the center →→ in the right hilum area. The right lower lobe is opaque, which indicates atelectasis caused by the tumor.

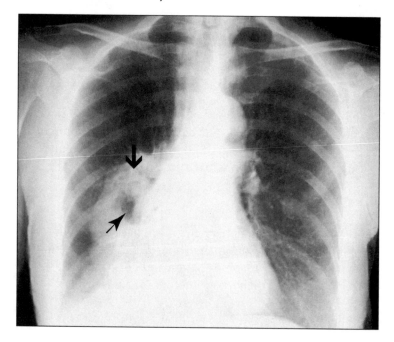

In large-cell cancer, the upper lung fields may appear to have a cavity.

Metastatic lung tumors usually occur secondary to primary GI, GU, and breast cancers. General symptoms are chest pain and nonproductive cough. Pleural effusion, elevation of diaphragm, and pleural masses with rib destruction may also be seen with metastasis. (See *Lung cancer*.)

⮑ Treatment

Surgical resection is usually the only hope for a cure. Unfortunately, detection is often late, well after metastasis has occurred. If the tumor can be resected, a lobectomy and, less often, a pneumonectomy, is usually performed.

Radiation therapy has varying effects, depending on the type of cancer. It can be a palliative approach to reduce cough, hemoptysis, bronchial obstruction, and superior vena cava syndrome.

Chemotherapy is used to treat nonresectable tumors, and it has increased the survival rate for some cancers. Long-term survival or cure is rare.

Pulmonary embolism

Pulmonary embolism is caused by obstruction of blood flow to the pulmonary arterial bed. The embolism may be a thrombus, tissue fragment, lipid, foreign body, or air. The most common cause is a thrombus that originates in the deep veins of the calf.

➟ Clinical signs

Most patients with pulmonary embolism have deep-vein thrombosis. They may also have leg swelling, duskiness, and Homan's sign (calf pain on palpation and dorsiflexion of the foot).However, most have no symptoms or signs involving the lower extremities.

Pulmonary embolism without infarct is the most common and the most difficult to evaluate. Signs and symptoms include tachycardia, tachypnea, dyspnea, unexplained anxiety, syncope, pleural pain, productive cough (possibly blood-tinged), low-grade fever, and pleural effusion. Less common signs include massive hemoptysis, splinting of the chest, leg edema and, with a large embolus, cyanosis, syncope, and distended neck veins.

In addition, pulmonary embolism may cause pleural friction rub, signs of circulatory collapse (such as a weak, rapid pulse and hypotension) and signs of hypoxia (for instance, restlessness). Pulmonary embolism with massive occlusion, profound shock, tachypnea, tachycardia, severe pulmonary hypertension, and chest pain indicates immminent death.

Chronic pulmonary emboli may lead to severe pulmonary

hypertension. Massive acute pulmonary emboli may cause shock and cardiopulmonary arrest.

⌣ Radiographic findings

Chest X-ray findings may not be helpful.
- Small areas of atelectasis or infiltration develop as surfactant is destroyed.
- Increased radiolucency distal to the embolism may be evident.
- Wedge-shaped infiltrates are characteristic.
- Pleural effusion may be present.

A $\dot{V}/\dot{Q}$ scan is ordered next. The scan identifies unperfused areas caused by the thrombus. The radiologist looks for a ventilation-perfusion mismatch on the study.
- Usually, the ventilation portion appears adequate.
- The perfusion portion has filling defects (the defining medium doesn't completely outline, or fill, the structure being examined), which indicates blocked pulmonary blood flow.

Pulmonary angiography is the definitive study for diagnosing pulmonary embolism. If the $\dot{V}/\dot{Q}$ scan is inconclusive and the diagnosis must be confirmed, a pulmonary angiogram will then be performed. It's the most invasive and most risky of diagnostic procedures. The benefits and risks should be explained to the patient and informed consent obtained by the radiologist prior to the study. Risks of the procedure include cardiac arrhythmias, reactions to the contrast, bleeding, and infection.

A pulmonary angiogram may show the following:
- filling defects in the artery
- an abruptly truncated (or cut off) vessel
- partial blockage of the pulmonary arterial branches, with an increased caliber proximal to the narrowing and a decreased caliber distal to the narrowing
- zones with deficient blood volume
- persistence of the dye in the proximal portion of the artery during the venous phase of the angiogram. (See *Pulmonary embolism,* page 55.)

To determine whether the patient has iliofemoral venous thrombotic disease, other diagnostic studies may be useful. These include Doppler ultrasound, contrast venography, and plethysmography.

⇨ Treatment

Treatment intends to maintain adequate cardiovascular and pulmonary functions during resolution of the arterial obstruction and to prevent recurrence of embolic episodes. Because most emboli largely resolve within 10 to 14 days, treatment consists of oxygen therapy, as needed, and anticoagulation with heparin to inhibit new thrombus formation. Heparin therapy is monitored by daily coagulation studies (partial thromboplastin time [PTT]).

Patients with massive pulmonary embolism and shock may require fibrinolytic therapy with urokinase, streptokinase, or alteplase to enhance fibrinolysis of the pulmonary emboli and remaining thrombi. Emboli that cause hypotension may require the administration of vasopressors. Treatment for septic emboli calls for antibiotic therapy, not anticoagulants, and evaluation for the infection's source, particularly endocarditis.

Surgery (pulmonary embolectomy) may be required. Vena cava filters may be inserted percutaneously if anticoagulant therapy is not successful or is contraindicated (such as in cerebrovascular accident, overt bleeding, or blood dyscrasias). The filters are placed above the renal veins to help catch clots before they reach the lungs. (See *Greenfield filter placement*, page 56.)

Surgery should not be done without angiographic demonstration of pulmonary embolism. To prevent postoperative venous thromboembolism, a combination of heparin and dihydroergotamine (Embolex) may be administered.

If the patient is receiving heparin, monitor coagulation studies daily. Effective heparin therapy raises PTT to approximately 2 to 2 ½ times normal. Watch closely for nosebleed, petechiae, and other signs of abnormal bleeding. Check stools for occult blood.

Pulmonary embolism

Left pulmonary angiography was performed for confirmation of pulmonary embolism prior to placement of an inferior vena cava filter. This image shows wedge-shaped infiltrate ➜, filling defects in the pulmonary artery and its bronchi ➤, and truncation of pulmonary artery branches ⟹.

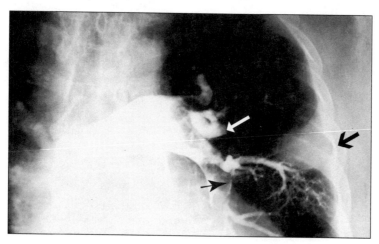

Most patients need treatment with an oral anticoagulant (warfarin) for 4 to 6 months after a pulmonary embolism. Advise these patients to watch for signs of bleeding, to take the prescribed medication exactly as ordered, and to avoid taking any additional medication or changing doses of medication without consulting their doctors. Stress the importance of follow-up laboratory tests (prothrombin time) to monitor anticoagulant therapy.

After the patient is stable, encourage him to move about often, and assist with isometric and range-of-motion exercises. Check pedal pulses, temperature, and color of feet to detect venostatis. Never vigorously massage the patient's legs.

Foreign bodies

Children and adults can aspirate a foreign body. In adults, partially chewed food, especially meat, is the most common aspi-

Greenfield filter placement

This abdominal X-ray was obtained after placement of a Greenfield inferior vena cava filter through the right internal jugular vein. Note the deployment sheath ➔. The filter is positioned with cranial tip ➤ just below the level of the renal veins.

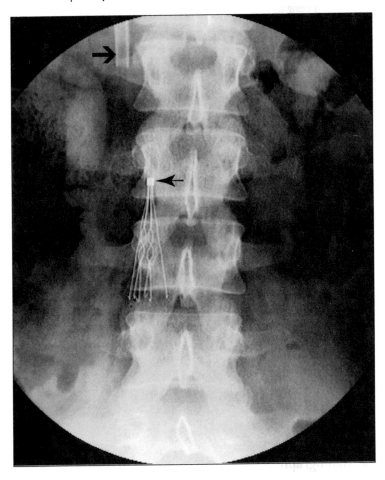

rate, with permanent dental work second. In children, a variety of small objects, including such foods as hot dogs or peanuts, may cause airway obstruction.

Foreign body

This is a classic inspiratory and expiratory anteroposterior chest X-ray of a 17-month-old with a ball-valve-type foreign body in the left bronchus. Inspiratory film is essentially normal, but expiratory film shows the left lung hyperinflated ➜ by the foreign body, because air is being trapped. You can also see a shift of the mediastinum to the right ➤ and relative increased lucency, or dark air-filled area, on the left.

INSPIRATION

EXPIRATION

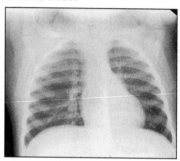 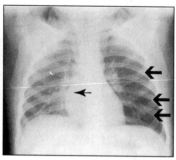

⭢ Clinical signs

Look for these signs of aspiration:
- inability to speak or cough forcefully
- vomitus or part of a foreign body visible in the mouth
- irregular, rapid, and shallow respirations (as the airway occludes) with slowly developing periods of apnea
- high-pitched inspiratory crowing or stridor
- expiratory wheezes
- cardiopulmonary arrest (possibly).

⭢ Radiographic findings

Plain X-ray films may reveal:
- a metallic object (coins or dental work) clearly shown on a chest film
- some nonmetallic objects shown as an opaque area with atelectasis or as an infiltrate distal to the foreign body

• the diaphragm, which won't rise on the side where the foreign body is lodged

• the diaphragm, which remains in the same location on inspiration and expiration PA chest films

• the heart, which may shift toward the obstructed side on inspiration and away from it on expiration. (See *Foreign body*, page 57.)

⮑ Treatment

Rapid removal of the foreign body is imperative if obstruction is complete. Perform an abdominal thrust in adults or chest and abdominal thrusts in children until the object is dislodged. If the item becomes lodged in the bronchus, bronchoscopy or surgery may be required to remove it.

Chest tubes and central lines

These devices allow doctors to remove air or fluids from the body, to feed patients, to administer chemotherapy drugs, and to obtain blood samples. Radiology provides a look inside the body to ensure proper placement of such instruments as chest or endotracheal (ET) tubes.

Chest tube

A chest tube may be as small as #5 French, or as large as #34, depending on its purpose. The tube is inserted percutaneously or surgically and may be made of vinyl, Silastic, or a non-thrombogenic latex material. It is inserted into the pleural space or mediastinum to remove air (pneumothorax) or to drain fluids (pleural effusions, hemothorax, empyema, or chylothorax), or to prevent air or fluid from reentering the pleural space.

After insertion, the chest tube will be connected to a negative-pressure setup (water seal, wall suction, or Heimlich valve) that will allow air and fluid to be expelled aseptically and that will also maintain negative pressure in the pleural space to keep the lung expanded.

➾ Radiographic findings

Note the following about X-ray findings.

• A pneumothorax in the apex of a lung will necessitate chest tube placement in an anterior upper lobe.

• Pleural fluid in the bases may require a larger bore chest tube inserted through a lateral chest-wall incision.

• The chest tube itself will be radiopaque or have a radiopaque line on it to facilitate viewing on the X-ray. The line should be straight, without any bends or kinks, and all holes (breaks in the radiopaque marker) should be within the rib cage.

• Comparing daily films will help determine whether the chest tube is dislodged and whether air or fluid drainage, or both, has progressed.

(For examples of chest tubes on chest X-rays, see *Pneumothorax*, page 39, and *Pneumothorax with subcutaneous emphysema*, page 40.)

ET tube

An ET tube is an artificial airway inserted into the trachea through the the mouth or nose. The tube may be cuffed (adult) or uncuffed (pediatric), and it has a radiopaque line extending along its length.

Indications for ET-tube insertion are:

• to ensure a patent airway
• to improve ventilation and oxygenation
• to control mechanical ventilation when required
• to administer anesthetic gases and medications
• to remove tracheobronchial secretions.

Equal breath sounds should be heard in both lungs on auscultation. External markings should be noted on the ET tube at insertion to maintain proper placement.

➾ Radiographic findings

• The end of the radiopaque marker should be 2 to 3 cm above the carina (bifurcation of the trachea into the right and left main bronchi).

• The clavicles are another reference point.
• The ET tube should be at the level of the clavicles if the clavicles are at the second or third rib.
• The cuff on the ET tube should be below the vocal cords. If a curve to the right is seen, the right mainstem bronchus may be intubated. The angle of the right bronchus is less sharp and is more commonly intubated. Likewise, a left curve means that the ET tube should be pulled back and repositioned.
• Note the position of the patient's head at the time of X-ray to determine correct positioning.

Central venous catheter

Central lines are increasingly used for I.V. administration of chemotherapy drugs, antibiotics, parenteral nutrition, and fluids. They are also useful in patients who require frequent blood sampling.

Doctors use the Seldinger technique to place standard central lines percutaneously. Longer-term lines are tunneled or implanted under the skin.

Hickman-type central lines have external access ports. An implanted infusion port (such as a PortaCath) has a site that can be accessed percutaneously with a non-coring needle.

All central lines are designed to deliver into central veins (generally the superior vena cava [SVC]) or the right atrium, where the vascular space is large and the blood volume is high. This minimizes venous injury caused by these often caustic agents.

⇨ Radiographic findings

The central venous catheter's placement should be confirmed by chest X-ray. On the X-ray, the catheter will appear as a line extending near the jaw into the SVC (if the internal jugular vein is used), or as a line running under the clavicle into the SVC (if the subclavian vein is used). A malpositioned catheter should be repositioned under fluoroscopy with the tip redirected down to the SVC.

If concern about placement remains, a small amount of

Repositioned central venous catheter
This fluoroscopic image shows the catheter has been repositioned with the tip at the junction of the superior vena cava and right atrium ⇒. A nasogastric tube can also be seen ➤.

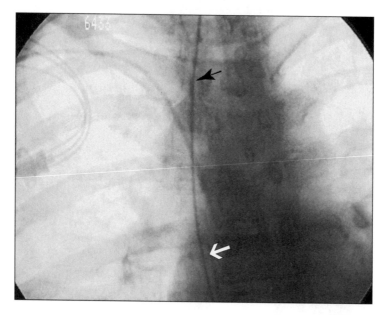

radiopaque contrast dye may be injected and films taken to verify position. When percutaneous subclavian lines are inserted, the chest X-ray should be examined for pneumothorax, which is a potential complication of catheter placement. (See *Repositioned central venous catheter.*)

Pulmonary artery catheter

A pulmonary artery catheter is a percutaneously inserted line, floated through the heart chambers and out into the pulmonary artery. Such a catheter is used to determine cardiac function by measuring the pulmonary artery pressure and the mean pulmonary artery wedge pressure (PAWP).

A small balloon at the catheter's tip is inflated to measure PAWP, which is a good indicator of left ventricular function.

Multiple tube placements

Note the various tube placements in this anteroposterior chest X-ray of a chest-trauma victim. An endotracheal tube ➜ is seen in the upper center portion of the picture. A nasogastric tube ⇾ can be seen as it passes into the stomach. A chest tube ⟹ is in place in the lower right side of the chest.

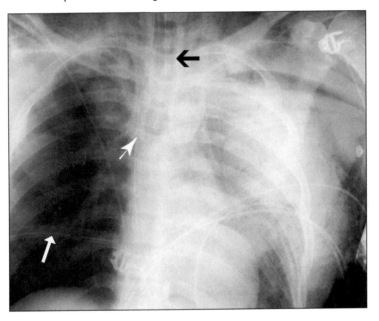

The balloon should be collapsed at all times, except when pressures are being measured, to prevent pulmonary infarction.

⇨ Radiographic findings

Insertion of a pulmonary artery catheter through the internal jugular or subclavian vein risks causing pneumothorax. Chest films should be closely examined for this. On the X-ray, the radiopaque line should follow the jaw (internal jugular) or clavicle (subclavian), go through the right atrium, the right ventricle, and out from the pulmonary artery with the tip in the distal branches to allow wedging.

Flail chest

This CT scan of the mid-chest region reveals rib fractures **A**, mediastinal emphysema **B**, subcutaneous emphysema **C**, and lung contusion **D**.

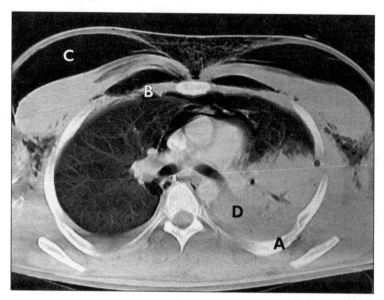

If the catheter is seen in the heart, report it because it should be repositioned to avoid arrhythmias. Knowing the appropriate waveforms and normal pulmonary-artery pressures will help determine catheter position.

Case study: Chest trauma

Mr. Venetti, a 22-year-old steelworker, was pinned to a wall by a 2-ton I-beam and sustained a sucking chest wound. He arrived in the emergency department (ED) with a penetrating injury of the right anterior chest, inferior to his right clavicle. He had been intubated at the scene. During transport, the ET tube became dislodged and entered his esophagus. He arrived in the ED with an SaO_2 of 55% and a stomach full of air.

The ED doctor ordered insertion of a right chest tube and

Repositioned right chest tube

This anteroposterior chest X-ray reveals a right chest tube repositioned into the upper pleural space ⇨. A left chest tube is evident in the lower pleura ➤.

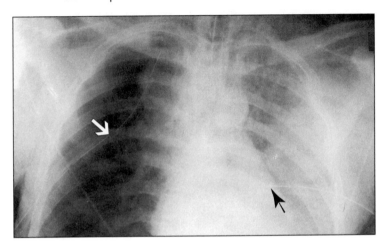

a nasogastric tube after the ET tube was repositioned. A bronchoscopy identified a blood clot in the right upper lobe of the lung. Vital signs after 10 minutes included a blood pressure of 177/58, a pulse of 101, and an SaO_2 of 91%. Mr. Venetti was stable enough to be transported to X-ray. (See *Multiple tube placements,* page 62.)

A CT scan revealed a flail chest with multiple left-rib fractures. (See *Flail chest,* page 63.) Further assessment showed the right-arm pulse decreased when compared with the left arm. A subclavian angiogram discovered an aberrant right subclavian arterial dissection. A right subclavian arterial stent reestablished blood flow to the right arm.

The next morning, Mr. Venetti remained in the intensive care unit in guarded condition. His chest X-ray showed a shift in the mediastinum to the right and a contusion of the left upper lobe. Subcutaneous air was seen in the soft tissue. A left chest tube was inserted, and 500 ml of blood was drained from the pleural cavity.

Resolving lung contusion

Note the resolving lung contusion ⇢ and marked overall improvement. Subcutaneous emphysema has resolved and tubes and lines have been removed.

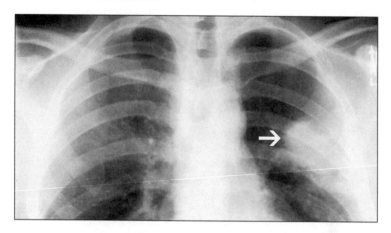

By noon on day 2, Mr. Venetti's condition had deteriorated into respiratory failure, and ARDS was diagnosed. Mechanical ventilation, I.V. fluids, and supportive measures were taken. A repeat CT scan showed the right chest tube had moved from its original position. It was reinserted into the right upper pleural space. (See *Repositioned right chest tube.*)

On day 6, Mr. Venetti's extreme pain led to shallow respiratory effort, resulting in atelectasis. The anesthesiologist inserted an epidural catheter to control thoracic pain. Then a vigorous pulmonary regimen was initiated.

On day 8, Mr. Venetti was extubated and able to breathe on his own. The next day, both chest tubes were removed and his status was much improved. A small right pneumothorax resolved itself without intervention. The epidural catheter was removed on day 13. On day 14, a chest X-ray was taken prior to Mr. Venetti's discharge. (See *Resolving lung contusion.*)

Mr. Venetti went home with orders for outpatient physical and occupational therapy. A CT scan taken 1 month later showed the lungs and ribs healing.

Guide to patient care

This chart outlines pretest and posttest care for respiratory system imaging technic

Test	Pretest care
Chest X-ray	• No food or fluid restrictions are required. • Remove jewelry from neck and chest and have patient don a gown. • Ensure that the female patient isn't pregnant.
Thoracic computed tomography scan	• No food or fluid restrictions are required if contrast medium isn't used. • Make sure the patient or responsible family member has signed a consent form. • If a contrast medium will be used, the patient should have no food or fluids for 4 hours before the examination. • Check the patient's history for hypersensitivity to iodine, shellfish, or radiographic contrast media. • If the patient is allergic to the contrast medium, provide appropriate pretest medication and hydration. • Remove jewelry from neck and chest. • Ensure that the female patient isn't pregnant.
Ventilation/perfusion (V̇/Q̇) scan	• No food or fluid restrictions are required. • On the test request slip, note whether the patient has conditions such as chronic obstructive pulmonary disease, vasculitis, pulmonary edema, tumor, sickle cell disease, or parasitic disease. • Determine if the patient has had any allergic reaction to radiopharmaceutical dye. • Remove jewelry from neck and chest.

Posttest care	Patient instruction
• None required	• Describe procedure. • Explain that he'll hold his breath briefly.
• Watch for delayed hypersensitivity to contrast medium (itching, hypotension or hypertension, or respiratory distress). • Encourage fluid intake, especially for patients allergic to contrast medium.	• Tell the patient he'll be positioned on a hard X-ray table that moves into the center of a large, ring-shaped piece of equipment; that the equipment may be noisy; and that the test may take 90 minutes. • Explain that a radiographic contrast medium may be injected into an arm vein. If so, explain that there may be nausea, flushing, or a salty taste. Reassure the patient with allergies that a nonionic medium will be used. • Tell the patient not to move during the procedure, but to breathe normally.
• If a hematoma develops at the injection site after the test apply warm soaks.	• Explain that a radiopharmaceutical will be injected into an arm vein and that the patient will sit in front of or lie under a camera. • Explain that neither the camera nor the uptake probe emits radiation. • Explain that the patient will be asked to briefly hold his breath after inhaling a gas and to remain still while the machine scans the chest.

Test	Pretest care
Pulmonary angiography	• Withhold food and fluids for 8 hours prior. • Make sure the patient or a responsible family member has signed a consent form. • Check the patient's history for hypersensitivity to anesthetics, iodine, seafood, or radiographic contrast media. • Ensure that the female patient isn't pregnant.
Ultrasonographic guidance for thoracentesis	• Withhold food and fluids for 4 hours before the procedure. • Ascertain whether the patient has an allergy to local anesthetics. • Have the patient or responsible family member sign a consent form.

Posttest care	**Patient instruction**
• Maintain a pressure dressing over the catheter insertion site. Note any bleeding. • Maintain bed rest for about 6 hours. • Watch for signs of myocardial perforation or rupture by monitoring vital signs. • Be alert for signs of acute renal failure such as sudden onset of oliguria. • Check catheter insertion site for inflammation or hematoma formation and report symptoms of delayed hypersensitivity response to the contrast medium or local anesthetic (dyspnea, itching, nausea, vomiting, tachycardia, or palpitations). • Encourage fluid intake and have patient resume his normal diet. • Advise patient about any activity restrictions	• Explain that a small catheter will be inserted into a blood vessel through a small incision and passed into the right side of the heart and into pulmonary artery. Dye will then be injected into the pulmonary artery and X-rays taken. • Explain that when the dye is injected, the patient may experience an urge to cough, a flushed feeling, nausea, or a salty taste for about 5 minutes. • Explain that heart rate and blood pressure will be monitored.
• Monitor the puncture site for signs of inflammation or infection (redness, swelling). • Monitor lung sounds, and respiratory rate and rhythm. • A chest X-ray is done after the procedure to assess for pneumothorax.	• Tell the patient to monitor the puncture site. • Explain that a chest X-ray will be done after the procedure.

Selected references

Dettenmeir, P.A. *Radiographic Assessment for Nurses*. St. Louis: Mosby–Year Book, Inc., 1995.

Laudicina, P. *Applied Pathology for Radiographers*. Philadelphia: W.B. Saunders Co., 1989.

Lewis, S.M, and Collier, I.C. *Medical Surgical Nursing: Assessment and Management of Clinical Problems*, 3rd ed. St. Louis: Mosby–Year Book, Inc., 1996.

Marieb, E.N. *Human Anatomy and Physiology*. Redwood City, Ca.: Benjamin/Cummings Publishing Co., Inc., 1989.

McCance, K.L., and Huether, S.E. *Pathophysiology: The Biologic Basis for Disease in Adults and Children*, 2nd ed. St. Louis: Mosby–Year Book, Inc., 1994.

Paul, L.W., and Juhl, J.H. *The Essentials of Roentgen Interpretation*, 3rd ed. New York: Harper & Row Publishers, 1972.

3 Cardiovascular system

The cardiovascular system delivers oxygen, nutrients, and other substances to all the body's cells and removes the waste products of metabolism. It performs this crucial task with blood, a vast network of veins and arteries, and the heart, which serves as the central pump.

Anatomy

The center of the cardiovascular system, the heart delivers blood throughout the body. A normal adult heart contracts at a rate of 60 to 100 beats a minute and pumps 5.5 L of blood through 60,000 miles (96,000 km) of blood vessels every minute.

The heart is a hollow, cone-shaped, muscular organ roughly the size of a fist. It's about 5" (13 cm) long and 3.5" (9 cm) wide and weighs between 9 and 13 oz (250 and 340 g), depending on a person's age, sex, and body size. In athletic young people, the heart may weigh slightly more than 12 oz; in elderly people, it may weigh slightly less than 9 oz. The heart lies within the mediastinum, a mass of tissue located between the lungs that encloses the heart and surrounding tissues. About two-thirds of the heart lies to the left of the body's midline. The bottom of the heart, or the apex, rests on the diaphragm. The top of the heart, or the base, is located just below the second rib.

Heart wall

A three-layer wall surrounds the heart. The inner layer, or endocardium, consists of a thin layer of endothelial tissue, which also lines the heart's valves and the chambers. The middle layer, the myocardium, is the thickest layer and consists of muscle tissues that contract to produce each heartbeat. The

Layers of the heart wall

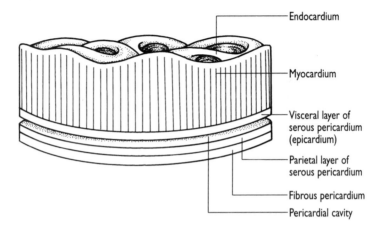

outermost layer, the epicardium, forms the inner layer of the pericardium, a sheath of tissue that encloses the heart and contains pericardial fluid. Pericardial fluid lubricates and protects the heart from friction. This inner layer of the pericardium is also known as the visceral layer of the serous pericardium. It contains the main coronary vessels, as well as the autonomic nerves, lymphatic channels, and fatty tissues. Between the visceral layer and the parietal layer of the serous pericardium is a thin film of serous fluid that holds the layers together, much as a thin film of water holds two microscope slides. The outside layer of the pericardium is known as the fibrous pericardium. (See *Layers of the heart wall.*)

Cardiac chambers

The heart has four chambers—two atria and two ventricles. The atria act as collectors for the ventricles, which produce the heart's pumping action. The right side of the heart receives blood from the systemic veins and propels it to the lungs, where it picks up oxygen and leaves behind carbon dioxide. The left side of the heart receives oxygenated blood from the pulmonary veins and pumps it into the systemic cir-

Cross section view of heart

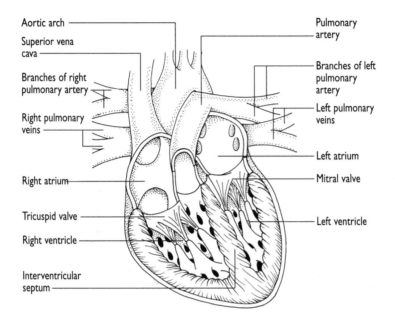

Aortic arch

Superior vena cava

Branches of right pulmonary artery

Right pulmonary veins

Right atrium

Tricuspid valve

Right ventricle

Interventricular septum

Pulmonary artery

Branches of left pulmonary artery

Left pulmonary veins

Left atrium

Mitral valve

Left ventricle

culation. The interatrial septum separates the right and left atria; the interventricular septum separates the right and left ventricles. The thickness of the walls in each chamber corresponds to the degree of high-pressure work performed by that chamber. The atria serve primarily as reservoirs and conduits for blood funneled into the ventricles, so their walls are relatively thin. Because the ventricles pump blood throughout the body, their walls are considerably thicker. The walls of the left ventricle are thicker than those of the right because the left ventricle pumps blood throughout the systemic circulation, whereas the right ventricle pumps blood only to the lungs. (See *Cross section view of heart.*)

Valves

Four cardiac valves allow blood flow through the heart in only one direction. The opening and closing of these valves depend on pressure gradients on both sides of them. Two atrioventricular (AV) valves—the tricuspid valve and the mitral or bicuspid valve—separate the atria from the ventricles, preventing a backflow of blood into the ventricles during ventricular contraction. The tricuspid valve, which has three triangular cusps, controls blood flow between the right atrium and the right ventricle. The mitral valve separates the left atrium from the left ventricle. Strong filaments called chordae tendineae attach the cusps of these valves to the ventricles' papillary muscles. The chordae tendineae and the papillary muscles stabilize the valves and prevent the valves' leaves from everting and allowing blood back into the ventricles. Dysfunctions of the chordae tendineae or papillary muscles can cause an incomplete closure of an AV valve, resulting in a murmur.

Known as the semilunar valves, the pulmonary and aortic valves each have three cuplike cusps, valves that open and close passively. The cusps respond to pressure changes caused by ventricular contraction and blood ejection. The pulmonary valve allows one-way blood flow from the right ventricle into the pulmonary artery. The aortic valve allows one-way blood flow from the left ventricle into the aorta. The closing of those two valves prevents backflow of blood into the ventricles.

Cardiac blood supply

The heart demands a constant source of oxygen. The coronary arteries and their branches supply the heart with oxygenated blood and metabolic substrates, while the cardiac veins remove carbon dioxide and other wastes from the bloodstream. When the heart's metabolic demands increase, coronary blood flow can increase to more than five times its resting amount. Because myocardial oxygen extraction stays fixed at about 65% to 70% of stroke volume enhanced coronary blood flow is the heart's only way of meeting its increased oxygen needs.

Coronary arteries

The right coronary artery and the left main coronary artery originate as a single branch of the ascending aorta. (See *Coronary blood vessels.*) The right coronary artery supplies

Coronary blood vessels

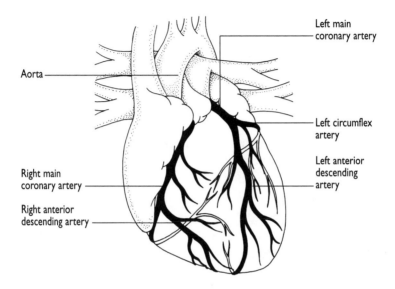

Left main coronary artery

Aorta

Left circumflex artery

Left anterior descending artery

Right main coronary artery

Right anterior descending artery

blood to the right atrium, right ventricle, and part of the inferior and posterior surfaces of the left ventricle. In most people, the right coronary artery supplies the sinoatrial (SA) node; in others, the circumflex artery supplies most of the blood to the SA node. The right coronary artery also supplies blood to a network of fibers called the bundle of His and to the AV node. The left main coronary artery runs along the surface of the left atrium, where it divides into two major branches: the left anterior descending (LAD) artery and the left circumflex artery.

The LAD artery descends toward the heart's apex. With its branches—the diagonal arteries and the septal perforators—the LAD artery supplies blood to the walls of both ventricles. The circumflex artery distributes oxygenated blood to the walls of the left ventricle and to the left atrium. The right coronary artery is often called the dominant artery—even though in most people, it is narrower and perfuses less of the myocardium than the left main coronary artery. The artery that crosses the crux (the point where the right and left AV grooves cross the posterior interatrial and interventricular grooves) is always referred to as the dominant artery. In most people, that vessel is the right coronary artery.

Coronary artery blood flow

During ventricular systole, the coronary arteries are squeezed, impeding blood flow. The coronary arteries receive blood primarily during ventricular diastole, when the aortic valve closes.

Whatever shortens the diastolic time, such as tachycardia, diminishes coronary artery blood flow. During bradycardia, diastole is prolonged, but coronary artery blood flow may be impeded by a lack of adequate pressure and by aortic recoil.

Cardiac veins

The thebesian veins, the anterior cardiac veins, and the coronary sinus and its tributaries drain blood from the myocardium into the right atrium. These cardiac veins run parallel to the coronary arteries.

Collateral circulation

When two or more arteries supply the same region, they usually connect with each other via anastomoses within the myocardium. Those anastomoses provide collateral circulation, or alternate blood routes. Typically, the myocardium contains numerous anastomoses connecting the branches of the coronary arteries. Collateral arteries may be present at birth, but they usually develop when oxygen demands change.

Conditions such as coronary artery disease, chronic myocardial hypoxia, and myocardial hypertrophy can cause collateral circulation to develop. Most collateral arteries in the heart are small. Blood from those arteries can keep heart muscle alive by supplying 10% to 15% of the organ's normal blood supply, the minimum required to prevent tissue death.

Conduction system

An electrical conduction system regulates myocardial contraction. This system includes the nerve fibers of the autonomic nervous system (ANS) and specialized nerves and fibers in the heart. The ANS involuntarily increases or decreases heart action to meet the individual's metabolic needs.

Both sympathetic and parasympathetic nerves participate in the control of cardiac function. With the body at rest, the parasympathetic nervous system controls the heart through branches of the vagus nerve. Heart rate and electrical impulse propagation are very slow. In times of activity or stress, the sympathetic nervous system takes control. It stimulates the heart's nerves to fire more rapidly and the ventricles to contract more forcefully.

Specialized pacemaker cells allow electrical impulse conduction. Pacemaker cells control heart rate and rhythm (a property known as automaticity). However, any myocardial muscle cell can control the rate and rhythm of contractions under certain circumstances.

SA node

Normally, the sinoatrial (SA) node (located on the endocardial surface of the right atrium, near the superior vena cava) paces the heart. Firing of the SA node causes impulses to spread throughout the right and left atria by way of internodal pathways, resulting in atrial contraction.

AV node

Impulses then travel through the AV node, which is located low in the septal wall of the right atrium, immediately above the coronary sinus opening. Normally, the AV node forms the only electrical connection between the atria and ventricles. The node initially slows the impulse, delaying ventricular activity and allowing blood to fill the ventricles from the atria.

Bundle of His and Purkinje fibers

Conduction then speeds through the AV node and the bundle of His. The bundle of His rises from the AV node and continues along the right intraventricular septum. It divides within the intraventricular septum to form the right and left bundle branches. Its fibers rapidly spread the impulse throughout both ventricles. Purkinje fibers, the distal portions of the left and right bundle branches, fan across the subendocardial surface of the ventricles, from the endocardium through the myocardium. As the impulse spreads throughout the conduction system, it prompts ventricular contraction.

Circulatory system

Through the circulatory system, blood carries oxygen and other nutrients to body cells and transports waste products for excretion. At specific sites on the body, the pressure of blood being pumped through arteries becomes palpable. The regular

Vessels of the circulatory system

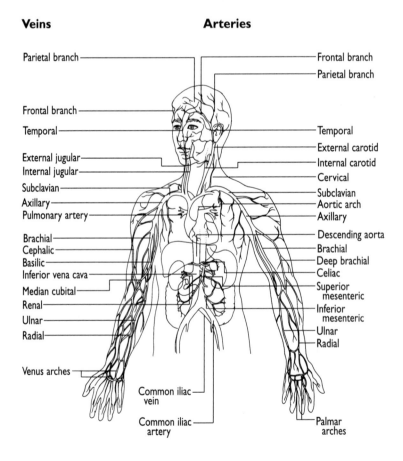

Veins

Parietal branch
Frontal branch
Temporal
External jugular
Internal jugular
Subclavian
Axillary
Pulmonary artery
Brachial
Cephalic
Basilic
Inferior vena cava
Median cubital
Renal
Ulnar
Radial
Venus arches
Common iliac vein
Common iliac artery

Arteries

Frontal branch
Parietal branch
Temporal
External carotid
Internal carotid
Cervical
Subclavian
Aortic arch
Axillary
Descending aorta
Brachial
Deep brachial
Celiac
Superior mesenteric
Inferior mesenteric
Ulnar
Radial
Palmar arches

expansion and contraction of the arteries is called a pulse. (See *Vessels of the circulatory system*.)

The body's major artery—the aorta—branches into vessels that supply specific organs and areas of the body. The left common carotid, the left subclavian, and the innominate arteries arise from the arch of the aorta and supply blood to the brain, arms, and upper chest. As the aorta descends through the thorax and abdomen, its branches supply GI and GU organs, the spinal column, and the lower chest and abdominal muscles. The aorta divides into the iliac arteries, which further divide into femoral arteries. (See "Case study: Systemic fibromuscular dysplasia," page 108.)

As the arteries divide into smaller and smaller units, called arterioles, the number of vessels increases dramatically, which in turn increases the area of perfusion. At the end of the arterioles and the beginning of the capillaries, strong sphincters control blood flow. Those sphincters can dilate to permit more flow through the capillaries, constrict to decrease flow and increase blood pressure, or close completely to shunt blood to other areas. Pressure within the capillary bed is normally low to permit exchange of oxygen and carbon dioxide with body cells. Blood flows from the capillary bed into venules (the smallest veins) and eventually into veins. Valves in veins prevent blood from flowing backward. The pumping action of surrounding muscles helps to return blood through the veins. Veins merge into larger and larger veins until they form two main veins, the superior and inferior vena cavae, that return blood to the right atrium.

Imaging techniques

Viewing heart and blood-vessel structure in detail allows radiologists to diagnose vascular conditions and to guide treatment. Vascular images of the heart and blood vessels are produced by using dyes that make vessels show up in crisp definition. That definition can be critical when planning treatment for hard-to-diagnose disorders. (For information about patient preparation and care, see *Guide to patient care*, page 112 to 119.) Here's a discussion of some of those imaging techniques.

Angiography

Angiography is the radiographic examination of one or more arteries or veins after injection of a contrast medium. When it's used to study arteries, the procedure is known as an arteriogram. When it's used to study veins, it's known as a venogram. In an arteriogram, a contrast medium is injected most often into the femoral artery; less frequently, the brachial or the carotid artery. Axillary or lumbar arteries may also be used.

Although indications for the test vary with the artery being studied, an arteriogram can provide information about blood-flow status, aneurysm formation, collateral circulation, vascular anomalies, tumors, and hemorrhage. Venography is often used to assess deep-leg veins. Lower-limb venography can confirm deep-vein thrombosis (DVT), identify causes of edema, and assess preoperative vascular status.

Angiography is invasive and it carries several risks—infection, vessel injury and occlusion, hematoma, bleeding at the puncture site, and allergic reactions to or renal toxicity from contrast materials. Radiologists weigh the risks against potential benefits and explain each to the patient before the patient signs an informed consent form. (See "Informed consent," page 7.)

Thallium scans

Also known as "cold spot" imaging, this test evaluates myocardial blood flow and myocardial cell status. Thallium scans can determine areas of ischemic myocardium and infarcted tissue and can evaluate the extent of pericardial effusion and of ventricular and coronary artery function. Thallium imaging can also detect an MI during its first few hours. Thallium-201, a radioactive isotope that emits gamma rays, closely resembles potassium. When injected I.V., the isotope enters healthy myocardial tissue rapidly but enters areas with poor blood flow and damaged cells more slowly. A camera counts the number of gamma rays given off by the cells and displays an image.

Areas with heavy isotope uptake appear light. Areas with poor uptake, cold spots, represent areas of reduced myocardial perfusion and appear dark. To distinguish normal from infarcted myocardial tissue, the doctor may order an exercise thallium scan followed by a resting perfusion scan. In an ischemic myocardium, the cold spot disappears—a reversible defect. In an infarcted myocardium, the cold spot remains— an irreversible defect.

Ultrasonography

Ultrasonography, a noninvasive procedure, uses high-frequency sound waves to reveal internal structures. When sound waves encounter a border or an interface between tissues, they bounce back to the source. A computer then evaluates this reflection, or echo, and displays the information on a screen.

Ultrasonography of the abdominal aorta can confirm an aortic aneurysm and is the preferred method for determining aneurysm diameter.

Echocardiography, a form of ultrasonography, records the reflection of ultrahigh-frequency sound waves directed at the heart. The test reveals heart size and shape, myocardial-wall thickness and motion, and valve structure and function. It also helps to evaluate left ventricular function and to detect mitral valve prolapse, cardiac tamponade, pericardial diseases, prosthetic valve function, ventricular aneurysm, cardiomyopathy, congenital defects, myocardial infarction complications, and valve insufficiency.

In transesophageal echocardiography, a transducer is placed in the esophagus next to the heart, allowing better visualization of the heart's anatomy.

Doppler ultrasonography

In this technique, a handheld transducer directs high-frequency sound waves to the vessel being tested. The waves strike blood cells moving through the vessel and bounce back to the transducer at frequencies that correlate to the speed of blood flow. The transducer amplifies the waves to permit direct listening and graphic recording of blood flow.

In a patient with a peripheral vascular disorder, Doppler ultrasonography can determine artery size and identify aneurysm location and size. The test is 80% to 90% accurate when used to detect DVT. In patients with varicose veins, it can quickly identify venous backflow.

Computed tomography

This test combines radiology and computer analysis of tissue density. In the procedure a series of tomograms is performed. A computer then translates the tomograms into an image on a screen showing details of a tissue cross-section. Vascular computed tomography (CT) scans are typically done to detail the location and the nature of aortic aneurysms.

Pathophysiology

Radiographic tests can help doctors diagnose a number of cardiovascular diseases and conditions that can affect the structure and function of the cardiovascular system. Patients who have the following diseases can expect to have one or more of the tests performed on them.

Coronary artery disease

Coronary artery disease (CAD) includes any vascular disorder that occludes one or more coronary arteries. Occlusion resulting from CAD can lead to diminished myocardial blood flow and decreased oxygen to myocardial tissues. Both of these conditions can cause ischemia. Either persistent ischemia or the complete occlusion of a coronary artery can cause infarction or cell death. (See *Coronary artery disease risk factors*, page 84.)

⇔ Clinical signs

The most common symptom of CAD is angina pectoris, or chest pain. Discomfort is usually transient, lasting 3 to 5 minutes. Angina pectoris is usually experienced as substernal chest pain that can radiate to the neck, lower jaw, abdomen, arm, or shoulder. Pallor, diaphoresis, dyspnea, and anxiety are usually present.

⮕ Radiographic findings

Accurate diagnosis of CAD, aided by sophisticated imaging methods, can prove lifesaving.
• Thallium imaging of the heart during or after exercise can show areas of decreased blood flow where coronary stenosis exists.
• To accurately assess perfusion, exercise must be sufficient to maintain 85% of the patient's maximum predicted heart rate. Images taken with the patient at rest are compared with images taken at peak exercise, when myocardial oxygen demand is greatest. Thallium scans can help confirm areas of ischemia in patients whose angiograms indicate possible stenosis.
• The most common angiographic finding in coronary artery disease is of one or more discrete stenoses, which may be long, focal, or occur in one or more vessels. Because many lesions are eccentric (one-sided), many different views may be necessary to accurately estimate the degree of stenosis.
• A less common finding of coronary atherosclerosis is ectasia (dilation) of the coronary arteries, which may appear as diffuse dilation or as a localized aneurysm. Prominent collateral circulation is frequently present when there is complete arterial occlusion but may also be present in severe stenosis. Collateral circulation may be present prior to obstruction and typically develops over several years of increasing occlusion. (See *Coronary artery stenoses*, page 85.)

⮕ Treatment

Coronary artery bypass grafting, the most common major surgery in the United States, is a popular way to treat CAD. In most of bypass operations, the saphenous vein or left internal mammary artery is used to bypass occluded coronary arteries. Long-term patency depends on such criteria as the patient's diet, blood pressure, smoking history, exercise, patient predilection for forming atherosclerotic plaques, and the surgical technique.

For some patients, the best treatment is percutaneous coronary artery angioplasty. A patient suffering from single-vessel disease with moderate to severe angina makes an ideal candidate for angioplasty. The success rate for this patient can exceed 90%. Multivessel angioplasty has greater risks and a lower success rate. Thrombolytic therapy may be used if large or numerous intracoronary thrombi are present.

Valvular heart disease

Valvular dysfunction may be the result of congenital or acquired damage caused by inflammation, ischemia, trauma, degeneration, or infection. Stenosis or incompetence may occur as a result of structural alterations of heart valves.

Valvular stenosis, a form of valvular dysfunction, can lead to valve-orifice constriction, which in turn impedes blood flow within the heart. The decreased blood flow increases the heart's workload.

Another form of valvular dysfunction, valvular incompetence or regurgitation, occurs when diseased cusps, or leaflets, fail to shut completely. Failure to close fully permits retrograde blood flow, which increases the volume of blood pumped by the heart and increases the workload of the atrium and ventricle. Ultimately, cardiomegaly and heart failure can occur. The valves of the left heart—the mitral and aortic—are affected more often by disease than are other heart valves.

Coronary artery disease risk factors

Nonmodifiable	Modifiable
Age	Hyperlipidemia
Male (until age 60)	Hypertension
Race (white)	Diabetes mellitus II
Genetic predisposition	Cigarette smoking
Diabetes mellitus I	Obesity
	Sedentary lifestyle
	Hormone therapy
	Heavy alcohol consumption

Coronary artery stenoses

This angiogram reveals coronary stenoses. The image in figure A reveals a high-grade stenosis of the right main coronary artery ➔. The image in figure B, taken from the same patient, shows high-grade stenosis of the left anterior descending coronary artery ➤.

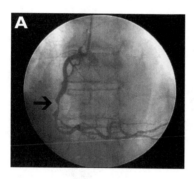
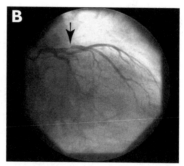

⮑ Clinical signs

The clinical signs of valvular heart disease are many and specific to the valves being considered. Some forms of valvular disease cause fatigue, dyspnea, orthopnea, palpitations, peripheral edema, syncope, chest pain, abnormal heart sounds, heart murmurs, and jugular vein distention.

⮑ Radiographic findings

• Heart valves may appear calcified on routine X-rays, which indicates valvular disease. However, valvular heart disease is best diagnosed by echocardiography or magnetic resonance imaging (MRI).

• A left ventriculogram shows thickened, poorly moving leaflets but no calcium in congenital aortic valve stenosis and regurgitation. When the stenosis is acquired, dense calcium appears in the valve and the anterolateral wall of the ascending aorta is dilated.

• Cine MRI, which produces moving images similar to those used in films, can detect evidence of aortic stenosis. Aortic valve leaflets appear thickened, calcified, and dark. Lack of proper flow during systole indicates aortic stenosis. (See *Heart valve replacement.*)

⇌ Treatment

Conservative treatment focuses on using antibiotics to prevent infection. Congestive heart failure is treated with digitalis, diuretics, and a low-sodium diet. Anticoagulant therapy is used to prevent and treat embolisms and to prevent clot formation in patients with atrial fibrillation. Nitrates may also be prescribed to increase coronary perfusion and cause peripheral vasodilation, which reduces the volume of blood returning to the heart and reduces the heart's workload.

Balloon valvuloplasty and valvulotomy may help patients with valvular stenosis when conservative treatment fails and surgery is not an option. Surgical repair or valve replacement is considered when other treatments fail or when symptoms appear when the patient is at rest. The type of surgery chosen depends on many factors, including the patient's age and life expectancy, ability to tolerate anticoagulant therapy, and type of valve to be repaired.

Conduction disorders that require pacemakers

Pacemakers assist or replace the heart's natural conduction system. Sometimes ventricles lack the necessary stimulus to contract as needed, a condition that warrants insertion of a ventricular pacemaker. Temporary pacemakers are used to treat a number of cardiac conditions and to restore electrical impulses in damaged cardiac muscles. Temporary pacemakers are inserted transvenously and have an external power source.

When continuous artificial pacing is required, a permanent pacemaker is surgically implanted. Permanent pacemakers, which have an implanted power source, may be unipolar (one lead) or bipolar (two leads) and may pace atria as well as ventricles.

Heart valve replacement

This lateral chest X-ray of a 57-year-old woman after heart-valve replacement surgery shows the porcine heart valve ➔. Note the pleural effusion ➤.

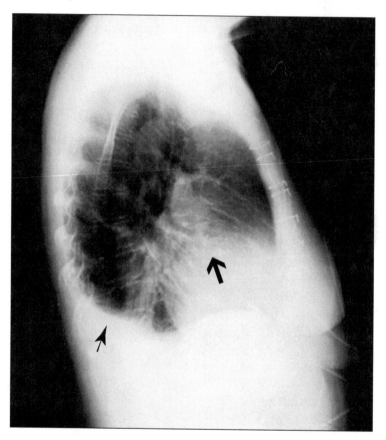

⮑ Clinical signs

Prior to pacemaker insertion, the patient may experience a variety of cardiac arrhythmias including bradycardia, supraventricular tachycardia, ventricular tachycardia, and asystole. The patient may also experience such symptoms as fatigue, syncope, palpitations, cyanosis, or malaise.

⮑ Radiographic findings

A chest X-ray after pacemaker insertion should reveal the
implanted energy source in the chest or abdomen, that the
lead wires aren't kinked or broken, and that they are in the
proper position. To ensure myocardial capture, the tip of a
temporary pacemaker should be imbedded firmly in the ventricular wall. (See *Pacemaker appearance on chest X-ray*, page 90.)

⮑ Treatment

Periodic chest films are used to check the location and condition of leads and wires. The films are especially important if
symptoms recur, a condition that may be caused by the pacemaker's failure to sense or to capture impulses.

Provide the patient with an identification card that lists the
pacemaker type and manufacturer, serial number, pacemaker
rate setting, date implanted, and the doctor's name. Watch for
signs of pacemaker malfunction and such complications as
infection, lead displacement, a perforated ventricle, cardiac
tamponade, lead fracture and disconnection, or Twiddler's syndrome. (This syndrome occurs if a pulse generator is too
mobile within the subcutaneous pocket and the patient twists
and turns it.) Teach the patient how to recognize the signs and
symptoms of these complications, and instruct him to notify
the doctor if any of these occur.

Carotid disease

Atherosclerosis of the carotid arteries can disrupt blood flow
to the brain, which may be permanent, leading to a cerebrovascular accident (CVA), commonly called a stroke, or
transient, causing a strokelike condition called transient
ischemic attack (TIA). TIAs are most often caused by thrombotic particles intermittently occluding cerebral circulation. A
true TIA is classified as one in which all neurologic deficits
resolve within 24 hours, with no residual dysfunction.

CVAs are classified as thrombotic, embolic, or hemorrhagic. Thrombotic strokes are caused by thrombi that occlude the

arteries that supply blood to the brain and intracranial vessels. The major causes of arterial thrombi are believed to be atherosclerosis and certain inflammatory diseases that damage arterial walls.

Embolic strokes stem from blockages caused by fragments of thrombi. The fragments, called emboli, break away from thrombi that have formed outside of the brain in the heart, aorta, carotid arteries, or other locations. These emboli obstruct vessels most often at narrowed junctions, which causes ischemia of tissues distal to the obstruction. Conditions that may precede an embolic event include atrial fibrillation, myocardial infarction, endocarditis, rheumatic heart disease, insertion of a valvular prosthesis, atrial-septal defects, and disorders of the aorta, carotids, or vertebral-basilar circulation. Air, lipids, and tumors can also cause embolic events, although less frequently.

Hemorrhagic stroke (intracranial hemorrhage) can be caused by hypertension, ruptured aneurysm, arteriovenous malformation, or by hemorrhage associated with bleeding disorders, particularly hypertensive hemorrhage in the brain.

➮ Clinical signs

Symptoms of carotid disease may vary depending on the location and extent of stenosis or thrombosis. TIAs may indicate a higher-than-normal risk of a future stroke.

Symptoms of TIA may range from visual disturbances (amaurosis fugax) to memory lapse, disorientation, hemiparesis, aphasia, and confusion. More severe stenosis or thrombosis can cause more destructive and lasting neurologic deficits including permanent hemiparesis, coma, and death.

➮ Radiographic findings

• Doppler ultrasonography of a stenotic carotid artery can show changes in waveform pattern and velocities, depending on the degree of stenosis. Stenoses can be categorized as mild, moderate, or severe, depending on waveform appearance and

Pacemaker appearance on chest X-ray

This posteroanterior (PA) chest X-ray of a 42-year-old woman with a pacemaker shows the battery ➜ and atrial ➤ and ventricular ➜ leads.

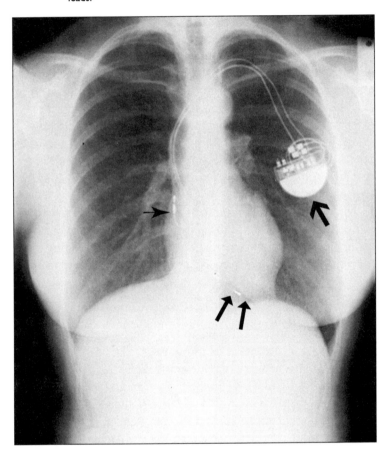

velocity measurements.

• Duplex ultrasonography may not differentiate between high-grade stenosis and total occlusion. For those determinations, angiography is often needed.

• An arteriogram of a diseased carotid artery may show the artery as tortuous, narrowed, or ulcerated. The most common sites of stenosis are the carotid bifurcation and the proximal portion of the internal carotid artery. Complete occlusion of the internal carotid artery generally indicates that surgery should not be performed. Selective catheterization of the carotid artery can show whether internal carotid artery flow is present. (See *Carotid selective angiogram,* page 93.)

⮑ Treatment

Treatment of carotid disease depends on the overall health of the patient. Embolic events are treated with anticoagulant therapy. Surgical intervention may be used to correct underlying disease conditions. Surgery is indicated if greater than 75% stenosis exists in an asymptomatic patient and greater than 50% stenosis exists in a symptomatic patient. Rehabilitative therapies are also indicated for patients with thrombotic or embolic strokes.

Disorders of the abdominal vasculature

Most disorders of abdominal vasculature—such as renal artery stenosis—are linked in some way to arteriosclerosis. Acute occlusion of the aorta or its principle branches may be caused by trauma, embolism, or thrombosis of a narrowed artery.

⮑ Clinical signs

Symptoms of these disorders depend on the arteries involved and the degree of involvement. Renal artery stenosis may cause a significant increase in blood pressure, as well as numerous other signs of renal disease. Stenosis of the mesenteric arteries may cause abdominal discomfort with digestion, along with weight loss and changes in bowel habits. Acute occlusion of any vessel can lead to ischemic changes in vessels distal to the occlusion. The most common signs of distal aortic occlusion include pain, loss of distal pulses, and color and temperature changes in the extremities. If left untreated, motor and sensory loss may occur.

⟿ Radiographic findings

Angiographic findings in patients with a diseased aorta
include the following.

• The aorta may appear irregular and tortuous from loss of
vessel-wall elasticity. The aorta may appear as if bites have
been taken out of it where plaques have formed.

• Vessels arising from the aorta—such as the celiac artery,
renal artery, superior mesenteric arteries, or inferior mesenteric
arteries—may appear narrow at their orifices.

• If the aorta is completely occluded, an abrupt termination
of the contrast column will appear. In such cases, distal structures will be filled by collateral circulation. (See *Aortic occlusion,*
page 94.)

⟿ Treatment

Treatment depends on the degree of involvement and symptoms and includes anticoagulant therapy, angioplasty, and surgical intervention. Acute ischemia requires rapid intervention
to prevent permanent tissue damage.

Peripheral vascular disease

Vascular disease of the legs is usually chronic and involves progressive narrowing and eventual obstruction of arteries that
supply blood to the legs. Peripheral vascular disease (PVD)
may affect the aortoiliac, femoral, popliteal, tibial, or peroneal
vessels. The disease is usually caused by atherosclerosis. By the
time symptoms occur, vessels may be more than 75% narrowed. The most common sites of involvement include the
femoral and popliteal arteries.

⟿ Clinical signs

The most common symptom of PVD is intermittent claudication, or pain in the muscles after exercise and relief at rest.
Peripheral pulses may be diminished or absent. Pain at rest
indicates insufficient blood flow to the skin and subcutaneous

Carotid selective angiogram

This film of a 52-year-old man shows disease in the common carotid bifurcation. There is a large ulcerated plaque ➔ and a 90% stenosis ➤ at the origin of the internal carotid artery.

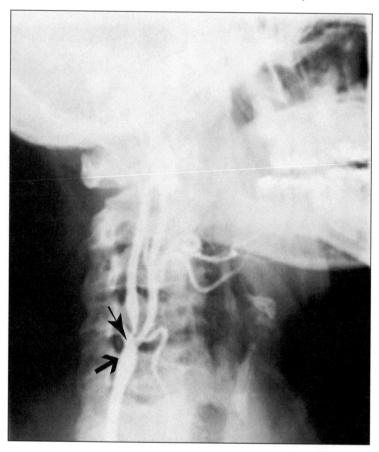

tissues. Without revascularization for those patients, ulceration and gangrenous necrosis eventually occur.

Paresthesia may result from ischemia of nerve tissue. Paling or blanching of the leg when raised indicates inadequate arterial flow. The skin becomes taut and shiny, and hair loss may occur.

Aortic occlusion
This aortogram is of a 59-year-old woman with a history of smoking who complained of pain in the buttocks and thighs. It shows aortic occlusion ➔ below the inferior mesenteric artery. Note the reconstituted iliac arteries filling by way of collateral circulation ➤.

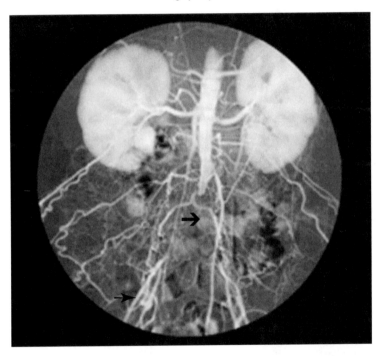

⤵ Radiographic findings

Aortography (angiography of the aorta) is the preferred technique for viewing branches of the aorta and vessels that supply the legs. Findings vary with the patient's anatomy. An aortogram may show calcification and blood vessel-wall irregularity.

• Filling defects and narrowings indicate the presence of atherosclerotic plaques that have invaded the vessel lumen.

• Diffuse vessel narrowing is a common finding, as is tortuosity and longer than normal arteries.

• Marked narrowing of a vessel can be easily missed on an

anteroposterior X-ray. Oblique views are required to assess
narrowed vessels. Careful assessment of gray areas and slightly
irregular segments increase the chances of locating lesions.

• The most common site of diseases in leg vessels is the
superficial femoral artery, particularly in the area of the adduc-
tor canal, a tissue tunnel in the middle of the thigh. Diabetic
patients have a higher incidence of stenosis and occlusion of
small distal arteries.

• If limb-salvage surgery is contemplated for a patient's
foot, the radiologist will pay particular attention to lateral
views. Lateral views are often needed to visualize and assess
the small vessels of the foot. (See *Focal, eccentric stenosis,* page
96.)

⇨ Treatment

Treatment depends on the severity of the disease and the progression of the patient's symptoms. The goals of conservative
therapy include protecting the limb from trauma, slowing disease progression, decreasing vasospasm, preventing and controlling infection, and improving collateral circulation.

More aggressive therapy is indicated if symptoms threaten
limb viability or incapacitate the patient. Treatment options
include surgical intervention by endarterectomy, bypass grafting, vascular stenting, or angioplasty. Saving the limb and
improving circulation are primary goals, as is improving the
quality of life for the patient.

Aneurysms

Aneurysms fall into three groups: true, false (or pseudo-
aneurysm), and dissecting. Each group and their associated
imaging techniques are discussed here in detail.

True aneurysms

A true aneurysm is a dilation, or outpouching, of the arterial
wall and is caused primarily by atherosclerosis. Plaques composed of cholesterol, fibrin, lipids, and other debris cling to

Focal, eccentric stenosis

Figure A is an angiographic image of a 49-year-old man with right-calf claudication. This bilateral leg angiogram reveals focal, eccentric stenosis of the right superficial femoral artery ⇒. Figures B and C are images from a series obtained during balloon angioplasty in the same patient. The image in figure B was made with the antegrade catheter positioned just above the lesion →. In figure C, you can see the guide wire and balloon catheter in place and the balloon → inflated to a diameter of 6 mm. The image in figure D was made after angioplasty. It shows a slight irregularity but no significant residual stenosis at the dilatation site →.

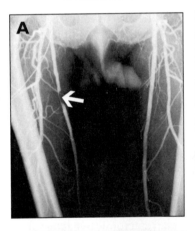

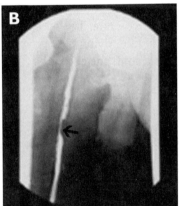

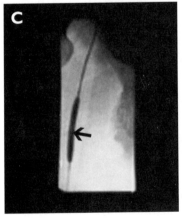

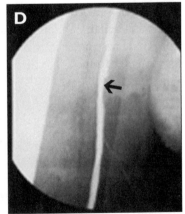

the vessel lining and cause degenerative changes, which then cause a loss of elasticity, tortuosity, and elongation of the vessel. Vessel-wall weakening can eventually cause dilation.

True aneurysms involve all three layers of the arterial wall, with at least one layer remaining intact. True aneurysms are further classified as fusiform, which have circumferential and uniform dilation, or saccular, which have eccentric (uneven) dilation. A saccular aneurysm has a narrow neck and is attached to the arterial wall. Causes of true aneurysms vary according to their location—thoracic, abdominal, or peripheral.

True thoracic aortic aneurysms. True aneurysms of the thoracic portion of the aorta—the ascending aorta and aortic arch—are rare. They may be associated with valvular disease or an underlying connective-tissue disorder. Aneurysms at the junction of the aortic arch and the descending aorta tend to develop spontaneously, most often from hypertension.

Aneurysms of the descending aorta tend to be of inflammatory, infectious, or atherosclerotic origin, and most arise at the terminal part of the descending aorta and continue to expand into the abdominal aorta.

True abdominal aortic aneurysms. Most true aneurysms are found in the abdominal portion of the aorta below the renal arteries, and usually occur in men over age 70. Most true aneurysms in the abdominal cavity are caused by atherosclerosis or, less often, by aortic dissection, vasculitis, infection, or trauma. The larger the aneurysm, the greater the chance of rupture. These aneurysms vary in size from a few centimeters in diameter to more than 10 cm. (The normal aorta measures 3 cm or less in diameter. Dilations of the aorta greater than 3 cm are considered aneurysms.) Half of all abdominal aneurysms more than 6 cm in diameter rupture within a year of diagnosis.

True peripheral aneurysms. Atherosclerosis is the most common cause of true peripheral aneurysms, which occur most often in the popliteal artery. These aneurysms are usually saccular and may be lined with mural thrombi, which form on an artery wall.

False aneurysms

A false aneurysm forms when a break in the arterial wall causes leakage of blood, which then compresses surrounding structures. False aneurysms are usually caused by blunt or penetrating trauma and can occur anywhere in the body. Causes of false aneurysms, like the causes of true aneurysms, vary according to their location.

False thoracic aortic aneurysms. These aneurysms are often caused by blunt trauma and usually result in a tear of the aorta adjacent to the origin of the left subclavian artery. The tear may cause rupture and death, but if bleeding is contained, a false aneurysm may form. Without prompt treatment, false aneurysms may rupture, a potentially fatal occurrence.

False abdominal aortic aneurysms. These aneurysms of the abdominal aorta are rare. They may arise from an anastomosis of a surgical bypass graft.

False peripheral aneurysms. False peripheral aneurysms may be caused by trauma, mycotic infection, or previous surgery. Postoperative aneurysms are often located at the anastomosis of a prosthetic graft and are usually saccular.

Dissecting aneurysms

A dissecting aneurysm (also called *dissection*) occurs when a tear develops in the intima of an artery. Blood exits through the tear and rapidly separates the inner from the outer layer of the arterial wall. Two lumens (a true and a false lumen) develop. Dissections may compromise normal blood flow and result in ischemic changes. They may also cause aneurysmal dilation or rupture and death. A dissection can develop in any artery from trauma or it can occur spontaneously.

Thoracic dissection. A vascular tear in the thoracic aorta may lead to a dissecting aneurysm. A dissecting thoracic aneurysm may be caused by trauma but frequently develops spontaneously as a result of atherosclerosis or hypertension or as a complication of systemic diseases such as Marfan's syndrome or fibromuscular dysplasia.

Abdominal dissection. Abdominal aortic dissections are usually extensions of a thoracic dissection. The abdominal aorta is rarely the original site of a dissection.

Peripheral dissection. Dissecting aneurysms of the peripheral vessels are usually caused by injury and can impair blood flow or prompt the formation of a thrombus.

⇔ Clinical signs

Clinical signs of an aneurysm depend on the type of aneurysms and its location.

True aneurysms

True thoracic aortic aneurysms. Most of these aneurysms are asymptomatic, but patients may complain of deep, diffuse chest pain. These aneurysms may also cause hoarseness from the pressure they exert on the recurrent laryngeal nerve. The patient may also experience dysphagia due to pressure on the esophagus.

True abdominal aortic aneurysms. Most of these aneurysms are asymptomatic until they enlarge and compress surrounding tissues. When symptoms do occur, they are usually caused by pressure on surrounding structures. Back pain may occur from lumbar-nerve compression. Epigastric discomfort with or without changes in bowel elimination may occur from bowel compression. A pulsatile mass may be felt in the periumbilical area. A bruit may be heard with a stethoscope over the aneurysm site.

True peripheral aneurysms. Common symptoms include pain at the aneurysm site, a palpable pulsatile mass, or swelling at the site. There may be diminished pulses distal to the site, due to decreased blood flow below the aneurysm.

False aneurysms

Signs of a false aneurysm are similar to those of a true aneurysm. Like a true aneurysm, a false aneurysm may be asymptomatic or cause only local signs and symptoms relating to pressure on surrounding structures.

Dissecting aneurysms

Thoracic dissection. The patient commonly complains of severe, sharp, tearing pain. If the ascending aorta is involved, the pain occurs in the right anterior chest or thorax; it may extend to the neck, shoulders, lower back, and abdomen. If the descending aorta is involved, the pain occurs between the shoulder blades and may radiate to the chest. Other findings may include pallor, diaphoresis, dyspnea, cyanosis, leg weakness, and neurologic changes.

Abdominal dissection. Because most abdominal dissections are extensions of thoracic dissections, expect the signs and symptoms described above.

Peripheral dissection. The most common findings are pain and neurologic impairments in the region of the dissection.

⮌ Radiographic findings

Findings of the various types of aneurysms, using different imaging techniques, are detailed below.

True aneurysms

True thoracic aortic aneurysm. An ascending or anterior aortic arch aneurysm can displace the trachea and esophagus to the left and posteriorly. The trachea and esophagus are generally displaced posteriorly by an aneurysm of the aortic arch and to the right and anteriorly by one of the descending aorta.

• The most common finding of a thoracic aortic aneurysm is a widened mediastinum on an AP chest X-ray. Linear calcification is often seen in the aneurysm wall.

• Aneurysms of the descending thoracic aorta usually occur to the left of the thoracic spine, as seen on the posteroanterior chest X-ray.

• CT scanning helps determine an aneurysm's origin and may reveal signs of aortic dilation and deformity, thickened aortic wall, mural thrombus, or calcification on the periphery or in the thrombus. CT scanning is also an effective tool for conducting follow-up studies after diagnosis.

• Aortography remains the diagnostic procedure of choice

for determining aortic branch involvement prior to surgical intervention. An aortogram may reveal a dilated aortic channel with peripheral irregularities, as a result of the aortic wall being thickened and atherosclerotic.

True abdominal aortic aneurysms. On AP and lateral abdominal X-rays, the presence of aortic-wall calcification may help diagnose an aneurysm. Significant calcification is present only half of the time, however, and other imaging techniques are better for diagnosis of these aneurysms.

• Ultrasonography is a safe, inexpensive, and reliable way of detecting and measuring abdominal aortic aneurysms. Its major drawbacks include difficulty in imaging obese patients and in potential imaging interference by bowel gas. The technique is also limited in detecting renal- or visceral-vessel involvement.

• CT scanning is highly accurate in finding true abdominal aneurysms and provides the only definitive assessment for ruptured aneurysms. (See *Pulsatile abdominal mass,* page 102.)

• Angiography is considered the method of choice for preoperative evaluation of the extent of involvement. Angiography also aids in choosing the appropriate surgical graft.

• Biplane aortography is necessary to assess aneurysm size and to evaluate visceral vessel origins. A lateral view helps show the aneurysm neck and the origins of the celiac artery and the superior and inferior mesenteric arteries.

• Pelvic arteriography is needed to show the extent of an aneurysm and the status of iliac and femoral arteries prior to graft placement.

Peripheral aneurysms. Ultrasonography is used to determine an aneurysm's size and shape. An intramural thrombus makes it difficult to assess size on arteriography. Prior to surgical intervention, note collateral involvement and the aneurysm's exact location. A lateral view is often needed to show the neck of a saccular aneurysm.

False aneurysms
False aneurysms often occur at prior graft sites or from traumatic tears.

Pulsatile abdominal mass

This image is from a lateral aortogram of a 64-year-old woman who presented with a pulsatile abdominal mass. The test reveals a focal, fusiform aneurysm of the abdominal aorta. Note the origin of the celiac →, superior mesenteric ➤, and renal ⟶ arteries. The aneurysm extends to just above the aortic bifurcation.

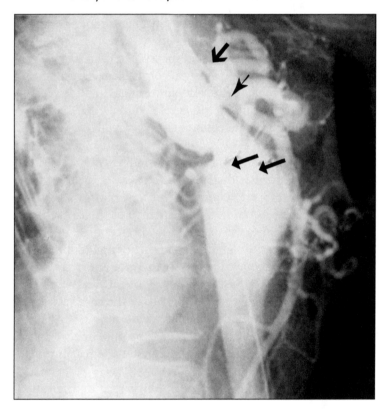

• On ultrasound or a CT scan, false aneurysms appear as vessel outpouchings and may be surrounded by thrombi.

• On an angiograph, false aneurysms are usually saccular in shape and have irregular contours.

Traumatic false aneurysms of the thoracic aorta usually occur immediately distal to the left subclavian artery. There may be an associated dissecting aneurysm, the mass may affect normal structures, and a left pleural effusion may be present. (See *Traumatic false aneurysm,* page 104.)

Dissecting aneurysms

In most cases of suspected dissecting aneurysm, speed and accuracy of diagnosis is essential.

• A widened mediastinum greater than 8 cm in diameter on chest X-ray may be the first indication of a thoracic injury and a possible aortic tear.

• Two-dimensional echocardiography can aid in the diagnosis of an ascending aortic dissecting aneurysm by showing a dilated aortic root, an oscillating intimal flap, and a so-called double-barreled aorta.

• CT scanning of the chest is often ordered to assess the integrity of the aortic arch and the descending aorta. The test may show the presence of a false lumen that may not become opaque during an angiography. Identifying the intimal flap is critical for diagnosing a dissecting aneurysm.

• An MRI scan may be used to visualize the intimal flap of a dissecting aneurysm and has the advantage of needing neither I.V. contrast dye nor ionizing radiation. In cine MRI, the intimal flap is outlined by bright blood flow through the true and false lumina.

• With angiography, the vessel wall may appear aneurysmal. Contrast material may also be seen below the adventitial layer of the vessel. Angiography can document ascending aortic involvement, aortic valve dysfunction, the locations of intimal tears, and the locations of sites of communication between true and false channels. Filling of branch vessels may also be seen. (See *Dissecting aneurysm in CT scan,* page 105.)

⇨ Treatment

Treatment varies with the type and location of the aneurysm.

True aneurysms

Thoracic aortic aneurysm. For long-term treatment, beta-adrenergic blockers and other agents can control hypertension

Traumatic false aneurysm

This is a lateral thoracic aortogram of a 32-year-old man who suffered multiple injuries in a motor vehicle accident. It shows an outpouching of contrast medium on the lesser curvature of the aortic arch distal to the left subclavian artery ⇒, indicating a traumatic false aneurysm. Note the origins of the brachiocephalic arteries ➤ and the incidental sinus in the aneurysm at lower left ➡.

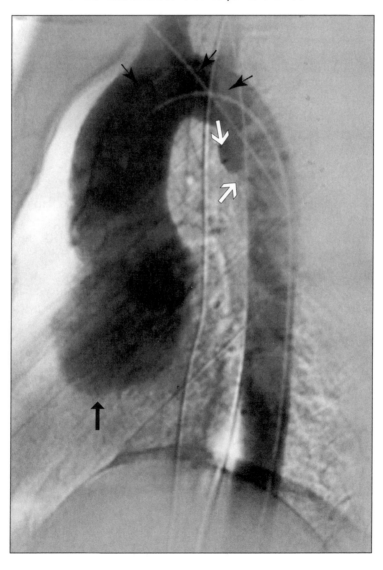

Dissecting aneurysm in CT scan

This CT scan, done at the level of the pulmonary artery bifurcation, is from a 66-year-old man who complained of chest pain that radiated to the spine. This image reveals a dissecting aneurysm of the descending thoracic aorta. Note the intimal flap ➔, and true ➔ and false ➡ lumens. Also shown are the ascending aorta **AA** and the superior vena cava **S**.

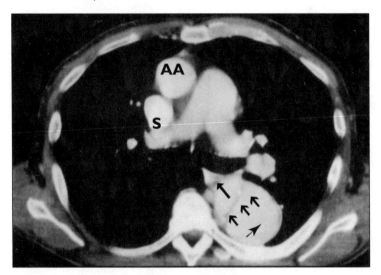

and cardiac output. In an emergency, antihypertensives such as nitroprusside, inotropic agents such as labetalol, oxygen, narcotic analgesics, and blood transfusions may be needed.

True abdominal aortic aneurysms. Surgical resection and grafting of the aorta remain the treatments of choice. The type of graft depends on the extent of aneurysmal involvement and the presence of other vascular diseases. A simple, tubular graft may be used if an aneurysm ends above the aortic bifurcation and if no significant iliac disease is present. An aortofemoral graft is used if disease is present in the iliac arteries.

True peripheral aneurysms. Surgical intervention is the treatment of choice and usually includes resection and graft.

Dissecting aneurysm in aortogram

This thoracic aortogram is of a patient with a dissecting aneurysm of the descending thoracic aorta. You can see the catheter ➔ in the true lumen ➤. Note the false lumen ➡ next to the true lumen of the aorta and the brachiocephalic vessels.

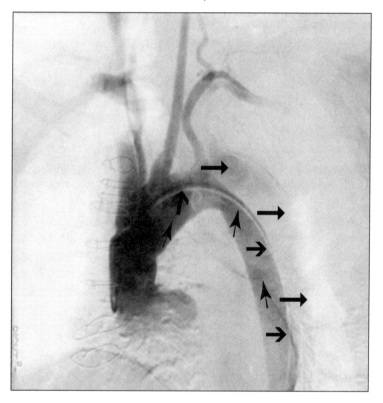

False aneurysms

Virtually all false aneurysms require treatment to avoid rupture and potentially catastrophic bleeding. Surgical repair is typically done. In some cases, nonsurgical intervention is the treatment. Use of covered-wall stents by way of percutaneous transluminal catheter angiography is gaining popularity as a nonsurgical means of repairing false aneurysms.

Dissecting aneurysms

The method of treatment often depends on the aneurysm's extent of dissection and on whether the ascending aorta is involved. Dissecting aneurysms of the ascending aorta are usually surgically repaired to reduce the risk of emboli formation, aortic valve incompetence, and tamponade. Patients who have uncomplicated dissecting aneurysms distal to the left subclavian artery may be treated conservatively. The aim of conservative treatment is to lower the blood pressure and reduce myocardial contractility, to diminish the force of aortic pulsations. (See *Dissecting aneurysm in aortogram.*)

Vascular trauma

Vascular trauma can stem from penetrating wounds, blunt trauma to overlying tissues, or numerous other injuries. Penetrating wounds may be caused by a bullet, a knife, or another penetrating object. Blunt trauma is a major source of injury in automobile accidents. For instance, ruptures of the aortic isthmus in a frontal collision in which the person isn't wearing a seat belt are common, as are tears in the lesser aortic curvature arch in broadside impacts. The main goal of diagnosing and treating vascular injuries is to expedite treatment before lasting damage or death can occur. Diagnostic studies establish indications for surgery. Because of the patient's grave condition, rapid diagnosis is critical. CT scanning is the method of choice for identifying vessel hematomas and parenchymal injuries in patients who have soft-tissue injuries. Angiography is the choice for more precise delineation of actual vessel injuries.

⇨ Clinical signs

Compression of an artery by edema or by other structures may displace a damaged artery or occlude it. Arterial spasm may be severe enough to cause decreased peripheral pulses. Pain at or near the injury site is common. Puncture wounds may cause edema and eventual ecchymosis and frank bleeding. Absence of peripheral pulses, decreased limb sensation, limb coolness, and lack of color in the limb indicate a disruption in blood flow.

⮎ Radiographic findings

- X-rays of an injured area often show soft-tissue edema along with other findings.
- An abdominal CT scan can help assess visceral injury or bleeding. There may be indirect evidence of a vascular injury, such as an aneurysm.
- Angiography is performed if any vessel tear, occlusion, or rupture is suspected. The vessel wall may appear aneurysmal or a collection of subadventitial contrast material may be seen, along with a tear in the vessel. In complete artery transection, a hook-shaped tapering may be seen. With arterial hemorrhage, contrast dye pools in surrounding tissues. If the vessel is small, it may go into spasm and temporarily stop bleeding, which could lead to an underestimation of the severity of injury.

⮎ Treatment

The usual treatment for an arterial tear, an occlusion, or a hemorrhage is surgical repair. If a patient's unstable condition prevents surgery, or if the bleeding site is accessible by percutaneous catheterization, angiographic embolization is recommended.

Case study: Systemic fibromuscular dysplasia

Mrs. Sanderson, 47, was diagnosed with systemic fibromuscular dysplasia (FMD) at age 42. FMD is a vascular disease that usually affects young adult women and is second only to atherosclerosis as a cause of renovascular hypertension. Mrs. Sanderson originally complained of headache, dizziness, and intermittent claudication of the right hip and thigh. Her

String-of-beads stenosis

This right common iliac angiogram shows a string-of-beads stenosis over several centimeters involving the external iliac artery ➔.

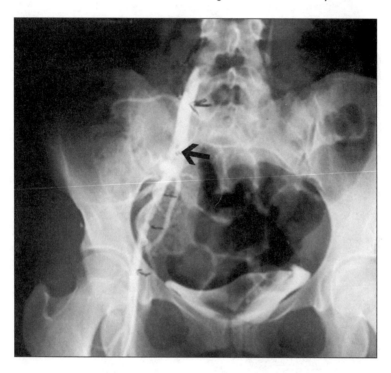

blood pressure averaged more than 200/110 at the time. Angiographic findings revealed evidence of FMD of both renal arteries and of the celiac artery, the superior mesenteric artery (SMA), and both iliac arteries. FMD stenosis involves hyperplasia of fibrin and of muscle cells within the media layer. Lesions may be focal, multifocal, tubular, or a mixture. Renal artery lesions usually affect the middle and distal portions of an artery; rarely the orifice. The classic radiographic sign of renal artery lesions is a string-of-beads appearance caused by alternating areas of narrowing and dilation in an artery that may be aneurysmal. (See *String-of-beads stenosis.*) A weblike fibrous band may appear inside the artery, which may

Early phase, lateral aortogram

This image, from the early phase of a lateral aortogram, shows no filling of the occluded celiac artery and a high-grade beaded stenosis of the proximal superior mesenteric artery →.

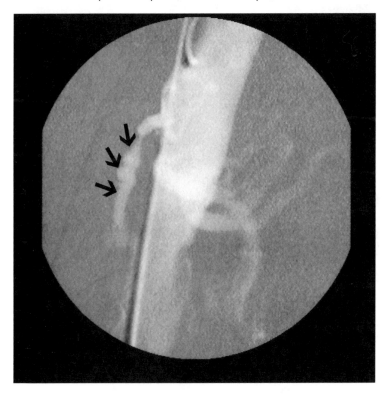

make it difficult to pass guide wires and catheters.

Mrs. Sanderson's doctors decided to treat her condition with balloon angioplasty. Because of the disease's complexity, only symptomatic areas were chosen for angioplasty. The procedure, angioplasty of the right iliac artery and both renal arteries, proved successful.

When Mrs. Sanderson's blood pressure rose again and her headaches returned, she underwent a right renal angioplasty. The procedure was successful. After discharge, she was monitored closely with ultrasonography and frequent blood-pressure checks. A year later, Mrs. Sanderson's headaches and dizziness returned.

A vascular study showed no noticeable difference in renal-artery status from films done the previous year. Her hypertension was treated conservatively with 2.5 mg of enalapril once a day.

A hypotensive crisis required her to be transferred to the intensive care unit, where I.V. fluids were rapidly administered and the enalapril dosage was reduced to 1.25 mg. She tolerated this adjustment well and was discharged in stable condition.

Fourteen months later, Mrs. Sanderson was readmitted for increasing abdominal pain consistent with atypical mesenteric angina. An aortogram revealed complete occlusion of the celiac artery and a high-grade (greater than 90%) stenosis of the proximal SMA. The stenosis was longer than 4 cm, the SMA was large, and a well-defined network of collateral circulation had formed. (See *Early phase, lateral aortogram.*)

With great difficulty, doctors catheterized and dilatated the SMA. The procedure established flow to numerous branches. The distal segment of the SMA also showed FMD, but doctors elected not to treat that segment at the time.

After angioplasty, Mrs. Sanderson noted some relief of symptoms but a small cramplike discomfort remained. Four weeks later in the clinic, Mrs. Sanderson described a marked decrease in abdominal discomfort. Her doctors continued to follow her condition.

Guide to patient care

This chart lists patient preparation and pretest and posttest care for various diagnostic-imaging tests of the cardiovascular system.

Test	Pretest care
Chest X-ray	• No food or fluid restrictions are required.
Abdominal aorta ultrasonography	• Instruct the patient to fast for 12 hours before the test to minimize bowel gas and motility.
Doppler ultrasonography	• No food or fluid restrictions are required.

Posttest care	Patient instruction
• No special posttest care is required.	• Explain that this test reveals the size and shape of the heart. • Instruct the patient to remove jewelry, other metal objects, and clothing above the waist, and to put on a hospital gown that has no metal snaps. • Explain that the patient may have to hold his breath while the film is being taken. • Check that the female patient isn't pregnant.
• Have the patient resume his usual diet.	• Explain to the patient that this test allows examination of the abdominal aorta. • Tell the patient who will perform the test and where. Explain that the lights may be lowered, that he will feel only slight pressure, that he must lie still and hold his breath periodically, and that the procedure usually lasts 30 to 45 minutes.
• Make sure to remove the conductive jelly from the patient's skin.	• Explain that this test is used to evaluate blood flow. • Explain that a blood pressure cuff is applied to the extremity to obtain accurate pressure readings and waveforms and that the patient will be asked to place his arms in various positions and perform breathing exercises as measurements are taken.

Test	Pretest care
Cardiac radiography	• No food or fluid restrictions are required.
Cardiac magnetic resonance imaging	• If the patient suffers from claustrophobia, he may require sedation before the test. • Have the patient void just before the test.
Lower limb venography	• Restrict food and drink to clear liquids only for 4 hours before the test. • Note any hypersensitivity to contrast medium on the patients chart.

Posttest care	Patient instruction
• No special posttest care is required.	• Explain that this test reveals the size, shape, and appearance of the heart and lungs. • Instruct the patient to remove jewelry, other metal objects, and clothing above the waist, and to put on a hospital gown without metal snaps. • Ensure that the female patient isn't pregnant.
• No special posttest care is required.	• Explain that this test assesses heart function and structure and may take up to 90 minutes to perform. • Inform patient that he will lie on a narrow bed that slides into a large cylinder. Explain that he will be able to communicate at all times and that the procedure will be stopped if he feels claustrophobic. • Instruct the patient to remove all metal objects. Patients who have pacemakers or a surgically implanted joint, pin, clip, valve, or pump containing metal won't be able to undergo the test.
• For 30 minutes after injection of a contrast medium, observe the patient closely for signs of anaphylaxis. • Monitor vital signs until stable. Check pulse rate using the *dorsalis pedis,* popliteal, and femoral arteries. • Watch for hematoma, redness, bleeding, or infection at the puncture site. • Instruct the patient to resume his usual diet and medication regimen.	• Explain that this test helps to detect abnormal conditions of leg veins. • Inform the patient that complications such as phlebitis and occasionally deep vein thrombosis can occur. • Warn that a burning sensation in leg upon injection of contrast medium or other discomfort during the procedure can occur. • Instruct the patient to remove all clothing below the waist and put on a hospital gown. • Explain that the test requires placement of a needle in the foot for contrast medium injection. • Instruct the patient to inform the technician immediately if he experiences dyspnea, nausea, severe burning or itching, or a constricted feeling in the throat or chest.

Test	Pretest care
Thallium scan	• Restrict alcohol and tobacco and the use of unprescribed medications for 24 hours before the test. • Restrict food and drink for 3 hours before the test.
Echocardiogrphy	• No food or fluid restrictions are required.
Transesophageal echocardiography with color flow Doppler	• Restrict food and fluids for 6 hours before the test. • Remove any dentures or oral prostheses, and note the presence of any loose teeth. • Connect the patient to a cardiac monitor, a blood pressure machine, and a pulse oximeter, and monitor all three during the procedure.

Posttest care	Patient instruction
• Have the patient resume his usual diet.	• Explain that this test helps to determine whether areas of the heart muscle are receiving adequate supplies of blood. • Inform the patient that he will receive an intravenous injection of a radioactive tracer, that images of his heart will be taken and that he must wear walking shoes during the treadmill exercise. • Instruct the patient to report fatigue, pain, or shortness of breath immediately.
• Make sure to remove conductive jelly from the patient's skin.	• Explain that this test is used to evaluate size, shape, and motion of various cardiac structures. • Inform the patient that he may be asked to inhale a gas with a slightly sweet odor (amyl nitrite) while changes in his heart function are recorded. • Describe possible effects of amyl nitrite (dizziness, flushing, tachycardia). Assure the patient that such symptoms almost always subside quickly. • Inform the patient he may be asked to lie on his left side, inhale and exhale slowly, hold his breath, or to inhale amyl nitrite.
• Keep the patient in the supine position until sedation wears off. • Whether lying supine or sitting upright, encourage the patient to cough after the procedure. • Restrict food and fluids until the patient's gag response returns. • Provide symptomatic treatment of the patient's sore throat.	• Explain that this test allows visual examination heart function and structures and the flow of blood through the heart's valves and vessels. • Inform the patient that an intravenous line will be inserted to administer a sedative before the procedure. • Explain to the patient that his throat may be sprayed with a topical anesthetic, that he may gag when the gastroscope is inserted, and that a block may be placed in his mouth so he doesn't bite the gastroscope.

Test	Pretest care
Cardiac catheterization	• Restrict food and fluids for at least 6 hours before the test but continue the patient's prescribed drug regimen unless directed otherwise. • Note any hypersensitivity to contrast medium on the patient's chart. • Have the patient void and put on a hospital gown just before the procedure.
Carotid arteriography	• Restrict food and fluids for at least 6 hours before the test but continue the patient's prescribed drug regimen unless directed otherwise. • Note any hypersensitivity to contrast medium on the patient's chart. • Have the patient put on a hospital gown and remove all jewelry, dentures, hairpins, and other radiopaque objects before the test.

Posttest care

- Monitor vital signs, skin color, temperature, and pulse distal to the puncture site every 15 minutes for the first hour after the procedure, then every hour until stable.
- Observe the insertion site for a hematoma or blood loss. Reinforce the pressure dressing as needed.
- If the femoral route was used for catheter insertion, enforce bedrest for 8 hours and keep the patient's leg extended for 6 to 8 hours. If the antecubital fossa was used, keep the patient's arm extended for at least 3 hours.
- Administer analgesics, as ordered.
- Check with the doctor about resuming the patient's diet and medications.
- Encourage the patient to drink fluids high in potassium such as orange juice. The potassium can counteract the diuretic effect of the contrast medium.

Patient instruction

- Explain that this test evaluates the function of the heart and its vessels.
- Inform the patient that he may receive a mild sedative but will remain conscious. Explain that he will be strapped to an X-ray table and that the table may be tilted to obtain different views of the heart.
- Advise the patient that the catheter used for imaging will be inserted into an artery or a vein in his arm or leg.
- Explain that he will experience a transient stinging sensation when a local anesthetic is injected prior to catheter insertion and that he may feel pressure as the catheter moves.
- Inform the patient that injection of a contrast medium through the catheter may produce a hot, flushing sensation or nausea that quickly passes.
- Assure the patient that if he experiences chest discomfort, he will be given pain medication and that complications such as myocardial infarction or thromboemboli are rare.

- Observe the insertion site for a hematoma or blood loss. Reinforce the pressure dressing as needed.
- If the femoral route was used for catheter insertion, enforce bedrest for 8 hours and keep the patient's leg extended for 6 to 8 hours. If the antecubital fossa was used, keep the arm extended for at least 3 hours.
- Administer analgesics, as ordered.
- Check with the doctor about resuming diet and medications.
- Encourage the patient to drink fluids high in potassium such as orange juice. The potassium can counteract the diuretic effect of the contrast medium.

- Explain that this test evaluates the quality of blood flow through the carotid arteries.
- Inform the patient that he will be positioned on an X-ray table with his head immobilized and that he should remain still.
- Describe possible adverse effects of contrast medium, such as a transient burning sensation as the medium is injected; a warm, flushed feeling, a transient headache, a salty taste, and nausea or vomiting.

Selected references

Dettenmeir, P.A. *Radiographic Assessment for Nurses.* St. Louis: Mosby–Year Book, Inc., 1995.

Diseases. Springhouse, Pa.: Springhouse Corp., 1993.

Laudicina, P. *Applied Pathology for Radiographers.* Philadelphia: W.B. Saunders Co., 1989.

Lewis, S.M., and Collier, I.C. *Medical-Surgical Nursing: Assessment and Management of Clinical Problems,* 4th ed. St. Louis: Mosby–Year Book, Inc., 1995.

Marieb, E.N. *Human Anatomy and Physiology,* 3rd ed. Redwood City, Ca.: Benjamin/Cummings Publishing Co., Inc., 1995.

McCance, K.L., and Huether, S.E. *Pathophysiology: The Biological Basis for Disease in Adults and Children,* 2nd ed. St. Louis: Mosby–Year Book, Inc., 1994.

Paul, L.W., and Juhl, J.H. *The Essentials of Roentgen Interpretation,* 3rd ed. New York: J.B. Lippincott Co., 1972.

Professional Handbook of Diagnostic Tests. Springhouse, Pa.: Springhouse Corp., 1995.

Taveras, J.M., and Ferrucci, J.T. *Radiology: Diagnosis-Imaging-Intervention,* vol. 4. Philadelphia: J.B. Lippincott Co., 1996.

4 Gastrointestinal system

The gastrointestinal (GI) system is responsible for ingesting and absorbing food, and for discarding wastes after useful food components have been absorbed. Specific radiographic tests can be used to evaluate conditions that hinder those functions.

Anatomy

The GI tract is a continuous, coiled, hollow muscular tube that winds through the ventral body cavity and is open to the external environment at both ends—the mouth and the anus. Organs of the system include the mouth, pharynx, esophagus, stomach, and the small and large intestines. The large intestine includes the anus. (See *GI tract anatomy*, page 122.)

The GI system digests food by breaking it down into fragments and absorbing those fragments into the bloodstream. Digestive activities include ingestion, propulsion, mechanical digestion, chemical digestion, absorption, and defecation.

Esophagus

The esophagus, a muscular tube that measures about 10" (25 cm) in length, is collapsed when not propelling food from the mouth to the stomach. The esophagus extends from the laryngopharynx to stomach, ending at the cardiac orifice. Along the way, it passes through the mediastinum of the thorax and the diaphragm, entering at the esophageal hiatus, where it joins the stomach. The gastroesophageal sphincter surrounds the lower end of the esophagus and acts as a valve to keep food in the stomach. The diaphragm, which surrounds the gastroesophageal sphincter, helps keep the sphincter closed when food is not being swallowed.

GI tract anatomy

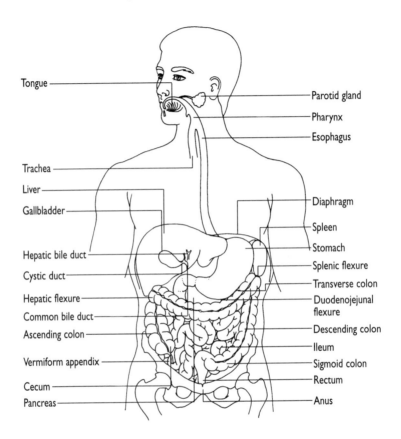

Tongue
Parotid gland
Pharynx
Esophagus
Trachea
Liver
Gallbladder
Diaphragm
Spleen
Stomach
Hepatic bile duct
Splenic flexure
Cystic duct
Transverse colon
Hepatic flexure
Duodenojejunal flexure
Common bile duct
Descending colon
Ascending colon
Ileum
Vermiform appendix
Sigmoid colon
Rectum
Cecum
Pancreas
Anus

Stomach

Below the esophagus, the GI tract expands to form the stomach, a temporary storage tank for food and an important site for mechanical and chemical breakdown. During this process, food is converted into a creamy, semifluid mass called chyme in preparation for its journey through the GI tract. (See *Stomach anatomy.*)

Normally, the stomach is a C-shaped mass located in the upper left quadrant of the abdominal cavity, where it's nearly hidden by the liver and the diaphragm. Although relatively

Stomach anatomy

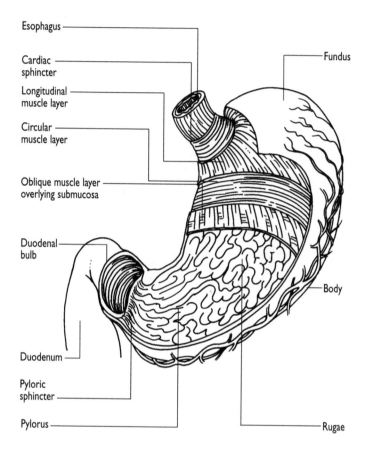

Esophagus

Cardiac
sphincter

Longitudinal
muscle layer

Circular
muscle layer

Oblique muscle layer
overlying submucosa

Duodenal
bulb

Duodenum

Pyloric
sphincter

Pylorus

Fundus

Body

Rugae

fixed at both ends, the stomach is somewhat moveable. Its location varies within the abdominal cavity. In short, obese people, for instance, the stomach tends to lie high and to run horizontally, giving rise to the term steer-horn stomach. In tall, thin people, the stomach tends to be elongated and to lie vertically within the abdomen, giving rise to the name J-shaped stomach. The stomach is usually about 10" (25 cm) in circumference but its diameter depends on how much food it contains. When empty, the stomach appears collapsed on itself, with its mucosa relaxed into large longitudinal folds called rugae.

The stomach consists of five major regions: the cardia, the fundus, the body, the antrum, and the pylorus. The cardiac region surrounds the cardiac orifice and is where food enters the stomach from the esophagus. The fundus is a bulge that lies superolaterally to the cardiac region. The body of the stomach is its middle portion. Between the body and the end of the stomach lies the antrum, where gastric acid is formed and which is a frequent site of disease. The pylorus, an area continuous with the small intestine and the pyloric sphincter, controls emptying of the stomach.

Small intestine

This twisted, hollow coil averages about 1" (2.5 cm) wide and is the body's major digestive organ. Within its convoluted passageways, usable food is prepared for the body's cells.

Digestion is completed in the small intestine with the help of secretions produced by the liver, the pancreas, and the small intestine itself. The small intestine, at a length of about 19.5' (6 m), is the longest section of the gastrointestinal tract. It extends in coils from the pyloric sphincter to the ileocecal valve and is encircled and framed by the large intestine.

The small intestine can be divided into three sections: the duodenum, the jejunum, and the ileum. The duodenum, which is about 10" (25 cm) long, curves around the head of the pancreas. Ducts that deliver bile from the liver and pancreatic juice from the pancreas join at the duodenum, at a common point called the hepatopancreatic ampulla.

The entry of bile and pancreatic juice into the duodenum is controlled by a muscular valve called Oddi's sphincter. The jejunum is about 8' (2.5 m) long and extends from the duodenum to the ileum, the most distal of the three small intestine subdivisions. The ileum is about 11.8' (3.6 m) long and joins the large intestine at the ileocecal valve.

Large intestine

The large intestine's major function is to remove water from indigestible food residue and to eliminate that residue as feces. The organ, which is about 5' (1.5 m) long, extends from the

Large intestine anatomy

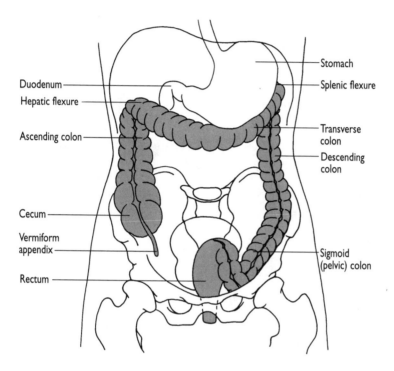

Stomach
Splenic flexure
Duodenum
Hepatic flexure
Transverse colon
Ascending colon
Descending colon
Cecum
Vermiform appendix
Sigmoid (pelvic) colon
Rectum

ileocecal valve to the anus. It frames the small intestine on three sides and is divided into the cecum; the ascending, transverse, and descending colon; the sigmoid colon; and the rectum. (See *Large intestine anatomy*.)

The saclike cecum, the first section of the large intestine, lies below the ileocecal valve. The vermiform appendix hangs from the cecum's inferior surface. The ascending colon lies vertically along the right side of the abdominal cavity and makes a right-angle turn, called the hepatic flexure. At that point, it becomes the transverse colon, which angles acutely at the splenic flexure. At that point, the transverse colon becomes the descending colon and lies vertically along the left side of the abdominal cavity. In the pelvis, the descending colon becomes the S-shaped sigmoid colon. At the level of S3, the sigmoid colon becomes the rectum, which runs inferiorly in front of the sacrum. The rectal terminus, or anal canal, ends at the anus, which has two sphincters—an inner involuntary one and an outer voluntary one.

Imaging techniques

A wide variety of imaging techniques are available to study GI disorders. Each technique requires its own patient-preparation protocol. Proper preparation of the patient is essential for obtaining high-quality images and reducing the risks associated with some of the tests. (For information on patient preparation and care, see *Guide to patient care,* page 166 to 171.)

Upper GI examination
An upper GI examination shows details of the mucosal lining of the GI tract and allows the radiologist to evaluate distensibility, to determine the status of extraepithelial layers, and to gather information about adjacent organs and structures. An upper GI requires that patients ingest a mixture of barium that outlines structures during imaging.

Double-contrast barium study
The double-contrast barium study uses gas (taken as carbon dioxide-producing granules) to distend the GI tract and barium to coat the mucosal lining. This study allows more detailed demonstration of mucosal morphology than a routine upper GI examination.

Nuclear medicine
In a nuclear-medicine study, the radiologist injects isotopes I.V. to identify problem areas within the GI tract. For instance, the test is used to find areas within the GI tract that are bleeding. The injected isotope "tags" red blood cells, while a scanner searches for pooled areas of the isotope.

Gastroesophageal reflux can also be diagnosed with nuclear studies. The patient ingests food or fluid laced with the isotope. The patient's esophagus is then scanned for evidence of the isotope after the point at which esophageal emptying should have occurred. Delayed emptying of the stomach can also be demonstrated with this technique.

Ultrasonography

Interference from bowel gas limits ultrasonography's usefulness in making images of the GI tract. But the test is highly useful in diagnosing appendicitis and pyloric stenosis in infants.

Computed tomography

Computed tomography (CT) scanning can prove highly useful in visualizing tumors, inflammation, herniations, perforations, and obstructions. A CT scan can also show cross sections of the GI tract and the surrounding anatomy with a single examination.

Angiography

This examination is used primarily to assess vascular anatomy in the gastrointestinal system. GI bleeding can be located and may be corrected through percutaneous embolization. Tumor vascularity may also be assessed by angiography prior to surgical resection. Mesenteric ischemia caused by vascular stenosis or occlusion may also be revealed and treated with balloon angioplasty. (See "Case Study: Small bowel obstruction," page 163.)

Pathophysiology

A number of diseases can affect the GI system and may require numerous imaging studies before a diagnosis can be made.

Esophagitis

The most common inflammatory condition affecting the esophagus is peptic disease, or reflux esophagitis. Other causes of esophagitis include Barrett's syndrome, scleroderma, naso-gastric (NG) tube irritation, infection (candidiasis, human immunodeficiency virus, tuberculosis, and fungal or herpetic infections), and a variety of other causes including radiation, Crohn's disease, effects of certain medications, and the inges-tion of caustic agents such as lye or bleach.

⟳ Clinical signs

Patients suffering from esophagitis usually complain of heart-burn. Other symptoms include chest pain, dysphagia, epigas-tric discomfort, and a choking feeling. Symptoms of reflux, or regurgitation of acid-bearing chyme, may also occur. Patients who have infectious esophagitis may notice oral lesions. Tet-racycline hydrochloride and potassium chloride tablets com-monly induce esophagitis. Other drugs known to cause esophageal inflammation include ascorbic acid, aspirin, doxy-cycline, ferrous sulfate, and quinidine.

⟳ Radiographic findings

Double-contrast barium techniques have greatly enhanced radiographic diagnosis of various types of esophagitis.
• Ulcer formation is the major finding of active esophagitis. These ulcers are usually linear and from 0.1" to 0.4" (3 to 10 mm) long, and are most often located in the distal esopha-gus. A radiolucent ring of edema may surround the ulcer.
• A thickening of the longitudinal folds of the esophagus may be seen. The folds may appear to have lobular or irregular contours. Mucosal nodules may also be seen.
• As the ulcers heal, scarring of the esophagus may be seen as a circumferential stricture in the distal esophagus.
• Abnormal motor function is common with severe inflam-matory changes, with peristaltic activity varying from minor dysfunctions to complete absence.

➥ Treatment

Esophagitis treatment depends on the cause of the inflammation. If acid is backing up from the stomach into the esophagus due to reflux, the doctor may order histamine blockers. (See "Reflux," page 150.) Metoclopramide, a smooth-muscle stimulant, may improve the functioning of the lower esophageal sphincter. Elevating the head of the patient's bed at night may aid healing. Drug-induced esophagitis is treated by discontinuing the offending agent. Susceptible patients can prevent the condition by taking their medications with plenty of water and by using medications that have an enteric coating. Severe scarring and stricture caused by chronic inflammation may require dilatation or surgical intervention.

Gastritis

Although stomach inflammation, or gastritis, can be caused by a wide variety of conditions, the most common cause is probably chronic or acute alcohol ingestion. Other causes include peptic ulcer disease, *Helicobacter pylori* infections, tumors, medications, Crohn's disease, and certain other less common conditions. Gastritis may lead to stomach-lining erosion and may be acute or chronic. Gastric erosion may be complete or incomplete, depending on whether the underlying condition has damaged the entire thickness of the mucosa or only part of it. Erosions greater than 0.2" (5 mm) in diameter are commonly referred to as ulcers.

➥ Clinical signs

Signs of acute gastritis include vague abdominal pain, epigastric tenderness, and GI bleeding. Chronic gastritis may not cause abdominal discomfort but may cause anorexia, fullness, nausea, vomiting, and epigastric pain. Bleeding may also occur.

Symptoms of a gastric ulcer include pain in the upper abdominal area, usually worse at night. Pain may be relieved with food or antacids. Anorexia, weight loss, vomiting, and bleeding may occur.

↩ Radiographic findings

Studies that reveal defects in soft-tissue structures can prove useful in diagnosing gastric ulcerations. Findings from X-ray studies using barium contrast include the following.

• Gastritis appears as mucosal erosions, thickened rugal folds, and poor stomach distensibility.

• Small erosions or ulcers may be seen as tiny flecks of barium that have a radiolucent halo of edematous mucosa. Larger, acute gastric ulcers may appear as defects in the mucosa with edema surrounding them. Those ulcers can also create round or oval puddles of barium.

Chronic ulcers create thickened margins that appear as smooth-surfaced filling defects around the ulcer. On profile view, chronic ulcers appear as conical or button-shaped projections extending from the gastric lumen. Rugal folds will radiate toward the ulcer. (See *Benign gastric ulcer.*)

↩ Treatment

Acute gastritis may heal spontaneously if the patient stops ingesting the agent that caused the condition, such as alcohol or aspirin. Antacids and histamine blockers help gastritis and ulcers heal by decreasing gastric-acid production. Antibiotics can be used to fight infections. Avoiding foods that cause discomfort also helps to heal the inflammation. For serious infections, surgery may be necessary if bleeding is severe and if conservative therapy fails.

Duodenitis

Duodenitis is an inflammation of the duodenum. The condition is often seen with peptic ulcer disease. Other causes of duodenal inflammation include pancreatitis, Crohn's disease, and certain infections, infiltrative conditions, and vascular disorders.

Duodenal ulcers are common and mostly affect the duodenal bulb. They occur more often in males than in females and are two to three times more common than gastric ulcers. Pan-

Benign gastric ulcer

This is a double-contrast study of a 74-year-old man's upper gastrointestinal system. He was experiencing epigastric pain and anemia. Note the ulcer crater ➔ on the lesser curvature of the stomach and the radiating folds ➤ .

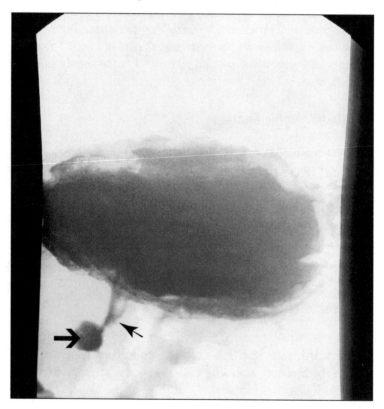

creatitis and cholecystitis can cause secondary inflammation of the duodenum, resulting in spasm and edematous folds.

Major complications of peptic ulcer disease include stomach obstruction, hemorrhage, duodenal bulb perforation, and penetration into and erosion of adjacent structures. Chronic postbulbar ulcers may result in a ring stricture (a chronic, progressive stricture that may lead to stenosis and partial or complete obstruction).

⇨ Clinical signs

Most inflammatory conditions of the duodenum produce intermittent upper abdominal pain. Symptoms are often temporarily relieved by food or antacids. Nocturnal discomfort as a result of acids pooling in the duodenum is common. The patient may experience a years-long pattern of remissions and exacerbations. Hemorrhage occurs in about 15% of patients and typically shows up as melena, occasionally as hematemesis.

⇨ Radiographic findings

When a small-bowel series, esophagogastroduodenoscopy, and upper GI tract X-rays are performed, major findings of duodenal disease include the following:
  • thickened folds, nodules, and erosions
  • small, round or oval ulcers, many with a radiolucent halo of edema surrounding them
  • a clover-leaf deformity of the duodenal bulb, a classic sign of healing chronic ulcer disease.

⇨ Treatment

Patients are usually treated first with antacids and histamine blockers. If hemorrhage has occurred, endoscopy is performed to find the bleeding site. The radiologist may attempt an angiography with selective embolization of the bleeding vessel. Arterial infusions of vasopressin are used to suppress acute, severe bleeding and to stabilize the patient's condition. Surgical resection is performed if conservative treatment fails.

Inflammatory bowel disease

Inflammatory bowel disease (IBD) is an idiopathic disease that may be caused by an immunologic response. Generally, two groups of IBD are recognized—ulcerative colitis and Crohn's disease. Features of the two groups often coexist, making diagnosis difficult. Both diseases occur more frequently in adolescents and young adults than in older patients, though periods of exacerbation may occur throughout the patient's life. The two groups will be discussed individually throughout this section.

Ulcerative colitis is usually confined to the bowel's mucosal and submucosal layers, with ulcers rarely penetrating into the muscular layer of the bowel wall. Typically, the bowel wall isn't thickened. The ulcers that occur in ulcerative colitis vary in size from patient to patient and are usually uniform within the same patient. Microscopic examination of ulcer tissues shows crypt abscesses and large inflamed cells. The disease is usually limited to the colon, with frequent rectal involvement.

Crohn's disease, by contrast, involves all layers of the bowel wall. Ulcers may vary in size, shape, and depth. The bowel wall and the adjacent mesentery may appear thickened. Entire sections of bowel may be unaffected, though effects of the disease may reappear in distal sections. In areas of extensive ulceration, the remaining inflamed mucosa is sometimes crisscrossed with deep fissures, a pattern referred to as *cobblestoning*. In many patients, cobblestoning may be found in the ileum and elsewhere in the GI tract. The bowel lumen is often narrowed in those cases and strictures can be seen. The colon may appear shortened and rigid, with fistulas in the most diseased segments. Noncaseating granulomas occur in 50% of patients.

⇔ Clinical signs

Though ulcerative colitis and Crohn's disease are manifestations of inflammatory bowel disease, they have different symptoms.

Ulcerative colitis
Patients usually experience fever, abdominal cramps, and bloody diarrhea. The onset of the disease is most often insidious, with periods of remission and exacerbation.

Other disease processes associated with ulcerative colitis include spondylitis, peripheral arthritis, iritis, certain skin disorders, and various liver abnormalities. Severe forms of ulcerative colitis may lead to hemorrhage, toxic megacolon, and cancer.

Crohn's disease

Symptoms of Crohn's disease include more intense and distressing diarrhea than that experienced in ulcerative colitis. Diarrhea in Crohn's disease is usually not grossly bloody. The crampy, colicky type of abdominal pain experienced by patients who have Crohn's disease is usually confined to the lower quadrants, particularly on the right side. Insidious weight loss from adjacent ileal disease may occur. Perianal or perirectal abnormalities occur in half of patients. There may be an increased risk of gallstones and renal calculi due to the effects of absorption abnormalities in the small bowel.

⟳ Radiographic findings

Ulcerative colitis and Crohn's disease cause distinctive radiographic findings used by the radiologist to help diagnose the diseases. Those findings include the following.

Ulcerative colitis

• Plain abdominal X-rays of patients suspected of having ulcerative colitis are used to rule out toxic megacolon or free intraperitoneal gas. (Those conditions preclude the use of barium enema, an imaging technique commonly used to diagnose ulcerative colitis and Crohn's disease.) Polypoid changes, large nodular protrusions of hyperplastic mucosa, and deep ulcers with intraluminal gas are all signs of ulcerative colitis.

• Barium-contrast studies early in the disease may reveal a hazy or fuzzy quality of the bowel contour, particularly in the rectosigmoid region. Those qualities stem from edema, excessive mucus formation, and tiny ulcerations of the tissue. Loss of haustral markings leaves folds flattened and squared off instead of rounded. The folds become thick, indistinct, and coarsely nodular. The thin coating of barium on the surface may appear stippled due to countless tiny ulcers, which cause

Toxic megacolon with ulcerative colitis

The 56-year-old woman from whom this X-ray was made complained of fever and abdominal pain and had an elevated white blood cell count. This abdominal film reveals a dilated, featureless colon with irregular, thick walls. Note the *thumbprinting* ➜ from wall edema and pseudopolyps ⤚▷ of edematous mucosa.

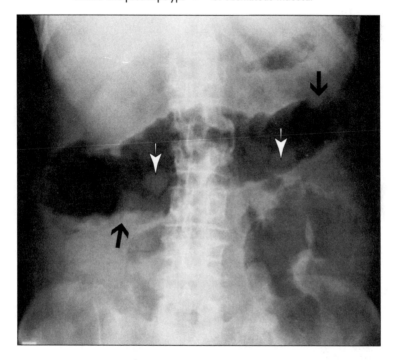

spike-like projections in a profile view. Progression of the disease leads to ulcerations of the submucosa and characteristic collar-button ulcers. (See *Toxic megacolon with ulcerative colitis.*)

Crohn's disease

• Small-bowel examination using barium contrast medium reveals tiny, discrete erosions (aphthoid ulcers) as pinpoint collections of barium surrounded by black radiolucent halos. As the disease progresses, the ulcers may deepen and become

more irregular. A great variety of sizes and shapes of ulcers can
be seen. Distribution of ulcers throughout the bowel is ran-
dom and asymmetric. A characteristic cobblestone appearance
of the mucosa is often seen.

• Penetration of the ulcers into adjacent structures can lead
to the formation of fistulas, which appear as a streak of contrast material outside of the bowel contours on X-ray. In late
stages, severe thickening of the folds can lead to a narrowing
of the lumen and stricture. (See *Crohn's disease.*) Pseudopolyps,
found in both types of IBD, are isolated areas of hyperplastic
inflamed mucosa between ulcerated areas. Pseudopolyps may
vary in size, shape, and pattern and usually appear as filling
defects in a section of bowel. Those defects may display a
nodular pattern.

⮎ Treatment

The treatment of both forms of inflammatory bowel disease
includes some of the same steps, but in all cases, therapeutic
regimens are tailored to meet the patient's individual needs.

Ulcerative colitis

Conservative treatment includes temporary dietary restrictions
to rest the bowel, controlling inflammation, combating infection, correcting malnutrition, providing symptomatic relief of
diarrhea and pain, and alleviating stress, which can aggravate
both conditions. Sulfasalazine and corticosteroids are considered
the drugs of choice for the treatment of ulcerative colitis. Surgical intervention is reserved for patients who fail to respond to
conservative therapy. Partial or total colectomy with ileostomy is
considered curative and alleviates the risk of colon cancer.

Crohn's disease

Treatment goals include controlling inflammation, relieving
symptoms, correcting metabolic and nutritional problems, and
promoting healing. Conservative treatment involves drug therapy and nutritional support. Sulfasalazine is effective when the
colon is involved. Corticosteroid therapy helps to reduce in-

Crohn's disease

This film was made during a barium examination of a small bowel. The 26-year-old woman had been experiencing abdominal pain and diarrhea. The X-ray reveals an edematous, thick-walled terminal ileum → with loss of normal folds and a contracted cecum →. Note the radiopaque ring →, a compression device used to enhance visibility of bowel-loop mobility and compressibility.

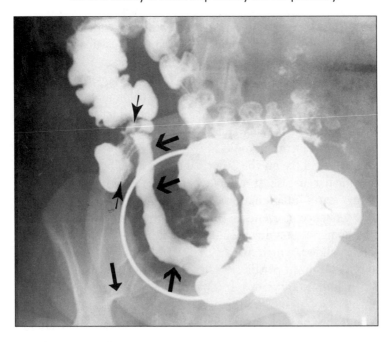

flammation. Total parenteral nutrition provides nutritional support during acute inflammation and after surgery, should surgery prove necessary. Dietary restrictions and use of an elemental diet can aid absorption. An elemental diet is a diet of residue-free, low-fat foods in a nutritionally-balanced meal. Foods used in an elemental diet are digested primarily in the upper jejunum. Surgery is not curative but may be necessary to relieve symptoms or to treat strictures if they're obstructing the bowel.

Diverticular disease

In diverticular disease, pouches form in the wall of the bowel. Those pouches can become inflamed and cause rectal bleeding. Occasionally that bleeding can be severe. Fistulas can form, and constipation alternating with diarrhea is common. This section discusses two common forms of diverticular disease—diverticulosis and diverticulitis.

Diverticulosis is a condition in which diverticula form within the bowel. Diverticula are saccular herniations of mucosa and submucosa that push through the muscular layers of the bowel wall. They can be found in as many as 50% of people over age 60. The sigmoid colon is most affected, perhaps because it has the smallest lumen of the colon and experiences the highest pressures within the GI system. That high pressure can cause the mucosa and submucosa to herniate through weak points of the sigmoid musculature and form diverticula.

Diverticulitis, on the other hand, is a complication of diverticular disease. It occurs when a perforation of a diverticulum creates inflammation or abscess of surrounding tissues. The sequence of events begins with entrapment of retained fecal material in a diverticulum. Inflammation of the mucosal lining follows, which may lead to perforation of the diverticulum. A localized peridiverticular abscess forms, usually walled off by fibrous adhesions. Intraperitoneal perforation may occur but does so rarely. An inflammation or an abscess may localize within the colon wall, producing an intramural mass, or it may surround the colon and cause a segmental narrowing of the lumen. The inflammatory process may spread to adjacent structures. Fistula formation is a common complication.

⮌ Clinical signs

Most patients with diverticulosis experience no symptoms. Those who experience symptoms often complain of chronic or intermittent lower abdominal pain, frequently brought on by or related to meals and emotional stress. Alternating bouts of constipation and diarrhea are common. A tender, palpable mass may be felt in the lower left quadrant. Painless bleeding, ranging from mild blood in the stool to massive hemorrhage, may occur. Patients who have acute diverticulitis often complain of left lower quadrant pain; fever; a tender, palpable mass; and an elevated white blood cell (WBC) count. If pericolic inflammation occurs, the patient may experience signs of bowel obstruction including constipation, nausea, anorexia, and abdominal distention.

➯ Radiographic findings

Diverticula appear radiographically as round or oval outpouchings of barium that project beyond the confines of the lumen. They may vary in size from dimples to saclike structures 0.8" (2 cm) in diameter. Usually multiple, they tend to occur in clusters. With multiple diverticula, a deep crisscrossing of thickened muscle can produce a sawtooth configuration. The involved section of colon may appear shortened and relatively fixed with a narrowed lumen. (See *Diverticula in descending and transverse colon,* page 140.)

Diverticulitis can be diagnosed radiographically through evidence of diverticular perforation.

• With a barium examination, the most specific finding is extravasation of contrast medium, which appears as a filled pericolic abscess or as a tiny streak of contrast coming out of the tip of the diverticulum. An extraluminal mass representing a walled-off perforation may appear as an extrinsic defect, causing an uneven narrowing of the bowel lumen.

• CT scanning is ideally suited for evaluation of diverticulitis. It can demonstrate thickness of the colonic wall and pericolic soft tissues. Multiple abscesses may appear as a single one that has a thick wall, with gas or fluid filling the lumen. Fistulas may appear as extraluminal collections of gas in the bladder, the vagina, or the abdominal wall. CT scans are also useful in guiding percutaneous discharge of diverticular abscesses.

Diverticula in descending and transverse colon

This is an oblique projection of a double-contrast barium enema. The 47-year-old woman presented with blood in her stools. The film shows scattered diverticula ➜ in the descending and transverse colon.

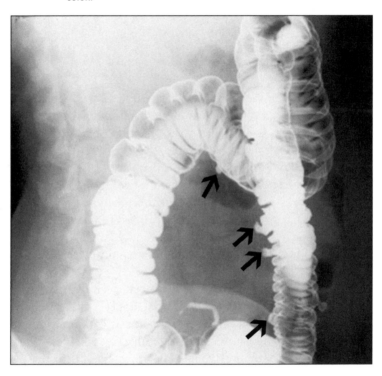

⤳ Treatment

Uncomplicated diverticular disease is generally treated with a bulk laxative and a high-fiber diet. Drugs such as dicyclomine or an antispasmodic-combination product, such as Donnatal or Kinesed, may be used to relieve bowel spasm. Acute diverticulitis requires antibiotic therapy. Bed rest, nothing by mouth, and the insertion of an NG tube may help to decrease bowel motility. Percutaneous drainage of an abscess using radiographic imaging may be performed prior to surgical intervention. In those cases, a bowel resection and a temporary diverting colostomy are usually performed.

Appendicitis

Appendicitis is an inflammation of the vermiform appendix, which lies inferior to the cecum. The most common cause of appendicitis is obstruction of the lumen. Lumen obstructions can be caused by a fecalith, a foreign body, intramural thickening, or a tumor of the cecum or appendix. If left untreated, obstruction may lead to gangrene or perforation of the appendix.

➮ Clinical signs

Periumbilical pain is often the first sign of appendicitis. Later symptoms include anorexia, nausea, vomiting, and a shifting of the pain from the periumbilical region to the right lower quadrant, coupled with rebound tenderness and muscle guarding. Low-grade fever and elevated WBC count are often seen. Complications of appendicitis include perforation, peritonitis, and abscess formation.

➮ Radiographic findings

• In ultrasonography, the appendix appears as a noncompressible, thick-walled, fluid-filled tubular structure that has no peristaltic activity. Echoes produced when soundwaves strike the appendiceal mucosa can appear as a bull's-eye pattern, with the edematous appendix wall forming the outer rings.

• On ultrasound, an abscess can appear as a mass next to the cecum or the appendix.

• On a CT scan, an inflamed appendix appears as a distended and fluid-filled, or collapsed tubular structure. Wall circumference thickens asymmetrically.

• Linear strands and haziness of the mesenteric fat on CT scans represent periappendiceal inflammation.

• Abscess formation may be seen as collections of pericecal fluid that have poorly defined margins or are encapsulated.

Postischemic stricture

This film is of a barium enema done on a 4-year-old boy who underwent multiple abdominal surgeries for injuries he suffered in a motor vehicle accident. He experienced abdominal pain and constipation. The film reveals a long postischemic stricture ➔ of the descending colon.

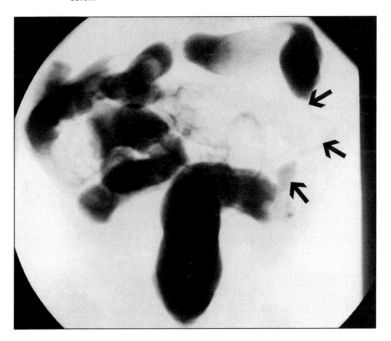

⮂ Treatment

If the appendix is intact, surgical resection is the treatment of choice. If rupture has occurred, conservative treatment with antibiotics, percutaneous drainage, nothing by mouth, and I.V. infusions may be used to treat peritonitis prior to surgical resection.

Strictures

Strictures of the GI tract may be caused by scar tissue left over from healing ulcerations, adhesions from previous surgery, or lesions of the bowel wall. Ischemias, tumors, medications, radiation therapy, chemical irritation from ingestion of caustic agents, anastomotic sites, and chronic inflammatory conditions such as Crohn's disease may also cause strictures.

⮆ Clinical signs

Signs of obstruction become evident as a stricture worsens and the lumen narrows. Depending on the site of the stricture, symptoms may include dysphagia, nausea, vomiting, abdominal pain and distension, bloating, decreased stool formation and, classically, hyperactive bowel sounds.

⮆ Radiographic findings

Although many imaging techniques are helpful in determining the specific cause of a patient's bowel obstruction, a CT scan is often the defining study.
• Contrast-dye studies show a tapered area of narrowing, with dilated bowel loops near the stricture. (See *Postischemic stricture.*)
• Contrast material may be completely missing distal to the stricture if the obstruction is complete. (See *Small-bowel obstruction*, page 144.)
• With pyloric strictures, the stomach may appear markedly distended. (See *Esophageal stricture*, page 145.)

⮆ Treatment

Dilatating the stricture with a balloon or with rubber dilators can be performed if the stricture is accessible by endoscopy or by a balloon catheter. Distal bowel strictures causing symptoms of obstruction may require surgical intervention.

Gastric-outlet obstruction

Peptic ulcer disease is the primary cause of gastric-outlet obstruction in adults. The obstructing lesion is often in the duodenum and occasionally in the pyloric channel or the

Small-bowel obstruction

A 73-year-old woman with breast cancer presented with abdominal pain and vomiting. A plain abdominal X-ray shows dilated, gas-filled bowel loops ⇒ and lack of colon gas, indicating a small-bowel obstruction.

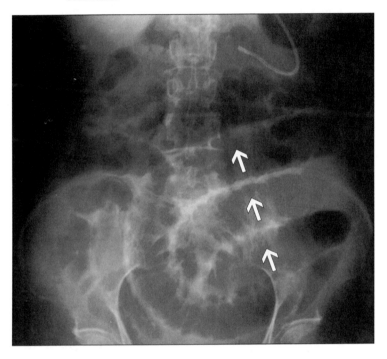

prepyloric antrum. Narrowing of the lumen may be caused by spasm, acute inflammation and edema, muscular hypertrophy, or contraction from scar tissue. Other causes of gastric-outlet obstruction include tumors, inflammatory conditions, congenital disorders, and previous surgery.

⇔ Clinical signs

Symptoms of gastric-outlet obstruction include epigastric pain and feelings of fullness. Eating may aggravate the pain; vomiting often relieves it.

Esophageal stricture

This is a lateral film of a 2-year-old boy with a history of lye ingestion and subsequent formation of an esophageal stricture. The film
was obtained during esophageal dilatation with a #27 French dilator
➔ across the stricture and into the gas-filled stomach ➤.

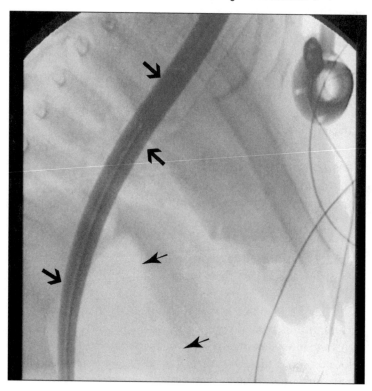

🔄 Radiographic findings

The main goal of radiologic examination is to tell whether
obstruction stems from a benign or malignant condition.

• Abdominal radiographs may show a large, shadowy outline of a distended stomach.

• Upright abdominal films may reveal a fuzzy, layered air-
fluid level different from the sharply defined air-fluid levels
normally seen in the bowel.

• Barium examination may show a mottled density of nonopaque material, which represents excessive gastric residue. The stomach may be large and may hang into the lower abdomen.

⮎ Treatment

Endoscopy is often needed to confirm the diagnosis and to biopsy the lesion. Medical management is similar to that used for ulcers and includes rest, stress reduction, and drugs to reduce inflammation. Pyloric balloon angioplasty may be useful in dilating strictures in benign cases. Surgical intervention may be required in severe cases.

Hernias and perforations

These conditions comprise a spectrum of disorders that can range in seriousness from irritating to life-threatening.

Hiatal hernia

Hiatal hernias, the most common diaphragmatic hernia found, are usually classified in three groups: sliding, paraesophageal, and mixed.

Sliding hernias account for more than 90% of all hiatal hernias. In this type of hernia, the esophagogastric junction forms the most proximal portion of the herniated stomach and is located above the diaphragm. The term *sliding* refers to the stomach's sliding through the hiatus when pressure in the abdominal cavity increases, and sliding back when the pressure decreases.

Paraesophageal hernias account for less than 5% of hiatal hernias. In those hernias, the esophagogastric junction remains below the hiatus but the stomach herniates into the chest, alongside the esophagus. There may be twisting of the herniated portion, which can cause strangulation.

Mixed hernias are a combination of the two types. A mixed hernia is often a large hernia with much of the stomach lying in the chest cavity.

↪ Clinical findings

Patients with sliding hiatal hernias may experience no symptoms. Those who have symptoms usually suffer from heartburn, regurgitation, abdominal pain, and dysphagia. Major complications of hiatal hernias include esophagitis, esophageal ulcers, and stenosis caused by cycles of fibrotic healing and scarring. Paraesophageal hernias usually don't cause symptoms of reflux, but the patient may experience such vague symptoms as postprandial indigestion, substernal fullness, nausea, occasional retching, and if the hernia is large, dyspnea after meals. The most frequent finding of a paraesophageal hernia is an ulcer at the point at which the stomach is compressed by the diaphragm. The most serious complication is gastric volvulus (twisting), which may lead to stomach incarceration and strangulation.

↪ Radiographic findings

Plain abdominal X-rays are used to detect hiatal hernias.
• Large hiatal hernias show up as soft-tissue masses in the posterior mediastinum. Those masses often appear with a prominent, layered air-and-fluid level.
• To diagnose a hiatal hernia, the esophagogastric junction must be well-defined and the diaphragmatic opening distinguished.
• Detection can be difficult unless a lower esophageal ring, or Schatzki's ring, is seen. Schatzki's ring appears as a thin, concentric, sphincter-like ring at the end of the esophagus, above the diaphragmatic hiatus. Detection of the ring implies that the junction is above the diaphragm and that a sliding hernia exists.
• The presence of obvious gastric folds, a mucosal notch, or a supradiaphragmatic pouch, without peristaltic activity and not in line with the esophagus, all suggest hiatal hernia. (See *Hiatal hernia,* page 149.)
• A paraesophageal hernia may protrude above the diaphragm and may appear as a pouchlike sac connected to

the esophagus. The hernia often appears as an air-fluid mass behind the cardiac silhouette.

Treatment

Treatment of hiatal hernia depends on the severity of symptoms. Surgical management is attempted in sliding hernias usually only if conservative treatment fails. Paraesophageal hernias with complications such as volvulus are managed surgically.

Perforations

Trauma or disease can cause the GI tract to perforate. Ingestion of a sharp-edged, foreign body may perforate the lining of the esophagus or other area in which the object is lodged. Esophageal dilatations and other treatments for esophageal stricture can rupture the lumen of the esophagus. Ulcerations that erode through a stricture wall can cause leaking of contents outside of the GI tract. Other diseases that can cause perforation include appendicitis, diverticulitis, bowel obstruction, and Crohn's disease.

Clinical signs

Symptoms of perforation include pain at the perforation site, abdominal tenderness or rigidity, fever, elevated WBC count, nausea, and decreased bowel sounds.

Radiographic findings

Plain X-rays, CT scanning, and contrast studies are used to determine the sites of perforation and to identify abscess formations.

• Free air in the peritoneal cavity on plain abdominal X-rays is a classic sign of perforation. Free air is seen as collections of air beneath the diaphragm.

• Contrast studies may indicate a perforation by showing a leak of contrast material outside of the GI tract. Gas patterns

Hiatal hernia

This upper gastrointestinal film of a 72-year-old woman shows a large hiatal hernia (the portion of the stomach above the diaphragm) ➔. Note the portion of the stomach below the diaphragm ➤.

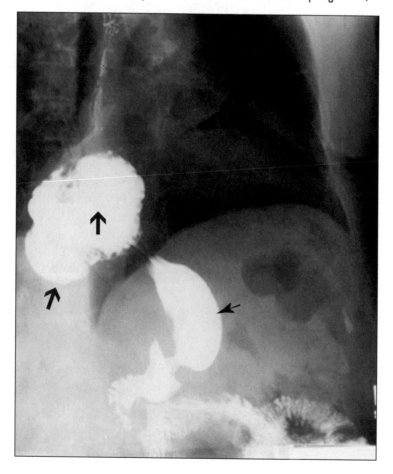

that may form inside abscess collections that occur postoperatively or as a result of a ruptured appendix or diverticulum are also visible.

• CT scans are performed to further localize abscess formation.

⏎ Treatment

Antibiotics and anti-inflammatory agents can aid the healing of a spontaneous rupture of the GI tract. Surgery is usually needed to resect a perforated bowel or appendix. Abscess formation may be treated by percutaneous drainage under radiologic guidance. This procedure is usually curative.

Reflux

Reflux esophagitis occurs when the lower esophageal sphincter (LES) fails to keep stomach contents from entering the distal esophagus. It is the main cause of esophageal ulceration and is frequently associated with hiatal hernia, though it may occur without it. Esophagitis may also be caused by prolonged vomiting. Reflux esophagitis commonly occurs in chalasia, a functional disturbance primarily seen in infants, in which the LES fails to remain closed between swallows. Failure of the LES to close allows regurgitation of large amounts of gastric contents into the esophagus. Patients who have scleroderma also may have a patulous LES, which predisposes those patients to reflux.

⏎ Clinical signs

Symptoms of reflux esophagitis are identical to those for esophagitis. (See "Esophagitis," page 127.) Patients who relate a history of regurgitating acid-tasting stomach contents probably suffer from severe reflux.

⏎ Radiographic findings

Determining reflux is generally not as important as identifying esophageal inflammation. Radiographic findings of reflux are identical to those of esophagitis.
• Applying a binder (which increases the patient's intra-abdominal pressure), having the patient perform Valsalva's maneuver, or having the patient lie in the Trendelenburg position may cause barium to be regurgitated into the esophagus.

Such barium regurgitation can help to identify reflux on imaging studies.

Treatment

Treatment for reflux is identical to that for esophagitis. Severe reflux can lead to an aspiration of stomach contents. Surgery may be needed to restore competency to the LES.

Adynamic ileus

Adynamic ileus occurs when fluid and gas don't progress normally through a nonobstructed small and large bowel. A variety of conditions predispose a patient to ileus, most commonly surgery, peritonitis, use of general anesthetics and other drugs, electrolyte imbalances, metabolic disorders, abdominal trauma, peritoneal hemorrhage, sepsis, shock, renal or ureteral calculi, mesenteric vascular occlusion, and certain neuromuscular disorders.

Clinical signs

A patient who has an ileus usually experiences abdominal distention, vague abdominal discomfort, and a marked decrease in bowel activity, which shows up as diminished bowel sounds.

Radiographic findings

Plain X-rays are most often used to diagnose ileus.
- An abdominal X-ray may reveal retention of large amounts of gas and fluid in a dilated small and large bowel.
- The entire small and large bowel are almost uniformly dilated. No point of obstruction can be seen.
- The stomach may appear distended.
- An isolated segment of distended bowel reflects a localized ileus and is often associated with an adjacent acute inflammatory process. The segment of bowel involved may provide clues to underlying diseases. (See *Ileus,* page 152.)

Ileus

The bowel-gas pattern in this 76-year-old man's postoperative abdominal X-ray reveals a diffuse, gas-filled dilation of the small bowel and colon, characteristic of an ileus.

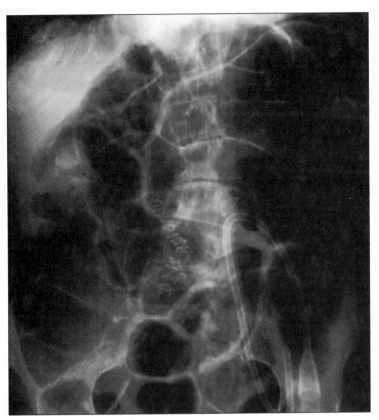

⟿ Treatment

Most patients respond well to insertion of an NG tube and I.V. fluids. The patient should receive nothing by mouth until active bowel sounds are heard. Correcting electrolyte imbalances and discontinuing offending medications may increase bowel activity. Patient mobility can increase muscle tone and speed the return of bowel activity.

Impactions

A fecal impaction is a large, firm, immovable mass of stool in the colon and rectum. It can develop when the patient is unable to completely evacuate feces over an extended time. Predisposing factors among adults include advanced age, immobility, debilitation, and the use of narcotics or large amounts of anti-anxiety agents.

➲ Clinical signs

Symptoms of fecal impaction include a vague rectal fullness and nonspecific abdominal discomfort. Overflow diarrhea—an uncontrollable passage of water and semiformed stool that occurs around a large impaction—commonly occurs.

➲ Radiographic findings

Several types of imaging techniques can reveal fecal impaction. Radiographic findings include the following:
  • A plain X-ray of the pelvis typically shows a soft-tissue density in the rectum. That density contains small, irregularly shaped, radiolucent areas that reflect the presence of gas pockets within the fecal mass.
  • Barium studies may reveal a large, irregularly shaped intraluminal mass.

➲ Treatment

Treatment for an impaction focuses on breaking up the stool such as with enemas and digital manipulation. Water-soluble contrast dye in enema may be used when an impaction is suspected of causing a large-bowel obstruction. The hypertonic solution draws fluid into the bowel to break up the stool.

Once the impaction is cleared, the goal of treatment is to prevent constipation and subsequent impaction. Measures may include increased fluid intake, dietary fiber, and activity.

GI tumors

Benign and malignant growths can occur in any part of the GI tract. Radiology is a key method for finding tumors and guiding treatment, which frequently involves radiation therapy. Early diagnosis often increases life expectancy.

Esophageal tumor

Cancer of the esophagus is relatively rare, accounting for 4% of GI malignancies. It strikes men more often than women and blacks more often than whites. Risk factors include excessive alcohol consumption and cigarette smoking. Other conditions associated with these tumors include achalasia, asbestosis, Barrett's syndrome, celiac disease, radiation therapy, oral and pharyngeal cancer, and excessive exposure to tannin.

⮑ Clinical signs

Progressive dysphagia is usually the first sign of an esophageal tumor. Mild substernal pain or fullness may be experienced. Regurgitation, hoarseness, and unexplained weight loss may also occur.

⮑ Radiographic findings

The radiologist will consider suspicious all tumors associated with abnormalities of the esophagus, including strictures, lesions, ulcers, and mucosal irregularities.

• Classic radiologic findings of esophageal tumors include the following patterns of tumor appearance: annular (apple-core), constrictive, polypoid, infiltrative, and ulcerative. More than one pattern may be present.

• Annular, or apple-core, lesions are the most common finding on X-rays. Those lesions have sharp, overhanging proximal and distal edges.

• CT scanning may be used for staging a tumor and for determining whether the tumor can be successfully resected. (See *Esophageal tumor*, page 156.)

⇨ Treatment

Early esophageal cancer limited to the mucosa or the submucosa and without lymph node involvement may be curable. Resection and radiation therapy is often successful.

Unfortunately, most esophageal cancers are found after the patient experiences symptoms of dysphagia, which signals infiltration of the malignancy and the presence of constricting lesions. Long-term prognosis in those cases is poor. Radical resection and reconstruction may be performed. In those cases, the stomach, jejunum, or colon is used to bridge the resected segment. Radiation therapy and palliative treatment may also be used.

Stomach tumors

Tumors of the stomach fall into four main groups: polyps, malignancies, submucosal tumors, and lymphomas. Most polyps are either benign or precancerous lesions. In early cancer, tumors are limited to the mucosa or submucosa. The patient's prognosis is good if his tumor is found early and treated appropriately.

⇨ Clinical signs

Clinical symptoms appear late in the disease and include anorexia, weight loss, malaise, and indigestion. Abdominal pain, vomiting, and a change in bowel habits occur later, as the disease progresses and metastasis occurs.

⇨ Radiographic findings

CT scans and plain X-rays can reveal stomach tumors.
• Polyps appear as filling defects that interrupt or displace the adjacent mucosa and gastric folds.
• In most cases, the remaining stomach mucosa appears atrophied.
• Early stomach cancer can appear as an elevation (tumor mass) or as a depression (ulceration).

Esophageal tumor

These chest-view CT scans were performed on an 81-year-old woman who presented with dysphagia and an esophageal mass. The study used oral and I.V. contrast. Figure A is a scan of the area just below the carina. Note the large soft tissue mass ⇒ in the dilated esophagus. Also seen in the image are the aorta **A**, the pulmonary artery **P**, and the superior vena cava **S**. Figure B shows an area of the chest about 4 cm below the area of the first image. Note the mass ➔ obliterating the esophageal lumen and compressing the left atrium. In figure C, in which the area right above the diaphragmatic hiatus, you can see the mass ⇒ and an adjacent large lymph node ⇢. Also apparent are the inferior vena cava **I** and the aorta **A**, and the left **LV** and right **RV** ventricles. In figure D, a scan of the upper abdomen, a lymph node mass ▶ is seen in the root of the mesenteric artery, just above the level of the celiac artery. Also note the spleen **SP**, liver **L**, kidneys **K**, inferior vena cava **I**, aorta **A**, and stomach **ST**.

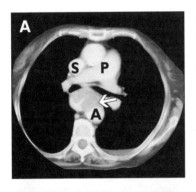

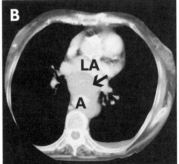

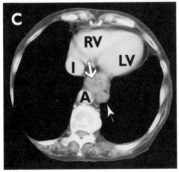

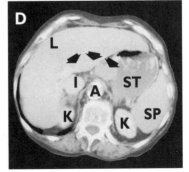

• Imaging studies of ulcerating cancers reveal irregular, saucer-shaped lesions with an ulcerated center.

• CT scans can often detect metastatic lesions, usually in the liver and the lymph nodes.

⮑ Treatment

Surgical resection of the tumor is the treatment of choice. Tumor staging and examining the patient for signs of metastatic lesions can help the doctor more accurately predict the patient's chance of survival. Chemotherapy may be used to shrink the tumor and to treat metastases.

Small-bowel tumors

The more distal the tumor is located in the small bowel, the greater is the risk of malignant disease. Adenocarcinomas make up the bulk of malignant tumors. Approximately 90% of duodenal-bulb tumors are benign.

⮑ Clinical signs

Benign tumors may ulcerate and cause acute or chronic GI bleeding and abdominal pain. Malignant tumors produce weight loss and anorexia and if located near the papilla, can cause obstructive jaundice. Bowel obstruction may develop.

⮑ Radiographic findings

CT scanning demonstrates the extent of primary disease and metastases and may guide needle biopsy.

• Benign tumors are usually discrete, smooth, and lobulated or polyplike. They may have ulcerated centers.

• Malignant tumors may appear as irregularly shaped ulcerations, nodular polypoid masses with overhanging edges, or destroyed mucosa with varying degrees of stricture formation.

⇨ Treatment

Surgical resection of the tumor is the treatment of choice unless staging reveals that the tumor can't be resected successfully. Chemotherapy may be used as a palliative measure.

Large-bowel tumors

Colorectal cancer is the second most common cause of cancer death in the United States. Adenocarcinoma of the colon occurs most often in patients between the ages of 50 and 70. Predisposing factors include villous polyps, ulcerative colitis, a family history of colorectal cancer, and high-fat diets without much fiber. Most large-bowel tumors spread through the bowel wall into the lymphatic system. Metastasis is common, and the 5-year survival rate is less than 50%.

⇨ Clinical signs

Most early colorectal cancers cause no symptoms. Right-sided colon cancers may produce symptoms of vague abdominal pain and weakness from iron-deficiency anemia, due to occult bleeding. Left-sided cancers often produce rectal bleeding, a change in bowel habits and stool appearance, and sensations of incomplete evacuation. Weight loss and cachexia are frequently seen when malignant tumors are present throughout the large bowel.

⇨ Radiographic findings

Radiographic findings of colorectal cancer include the following.

• In barium enemas studies, annular carcinomas typically appear as apple-core lesions. The narrowed segment is usually short and has sharply defined edges. Normal mucosal detail is destroyed.

• CT scanning may be helpful in staging the tumor and in finding metastatic lesions.

• On CT scans, there may be thickening of the bowel wall

and narrowing and deformity of the lumen. (See *Apple-core lesion,* page 160.)

↝ Treatment

Treatment and prognosis depend on the stage of tumor growth. Surgical resection is the treatment of choice for most tumors, and a colostomy is often necessary. Radiation therapy and chemotherapy may be used to manage metastatic disease and to reduce symptoms of metastasis.

Foreign bodies

A foreign body is an object ingested or inserted into the GI tract that lodges in the lumen or penetrates the alimentary-canal wall. Examples of foreign bodies include toys, poorly chewed food (usually meat), or fish or chicken bones swallowed accidentally.

Children may swallow any object small enough to fit into their mouths. Metal toys or other metal objects may be evident on X-rays. Plastic or light alloys may prove much more difficult to see.

↝ Clinical signs

Signs of obstruction may occur if a foreign body occludes the lumen of a section of the GI tract. Complications of esophageal foreign bodies may include penetration, which could cause periesophageal abscess or diffuse mediastinitis. Peritonitis can develop following intestinal perforations. Dysphagia, stridor, or recurrent pneumonia may occur in children not known to have ingested a foreign body.

↝ Radiographic findings

Multiple views of objects are often necessary to determine whether a foreign body lies within the lumen and is obstructing flow. (See *Foreign body,* page 161.)

Apple-core lesion

This barium enema in a 61-year-old patient shows a classic apple core lesion ⇒ at the hepatic flexure.

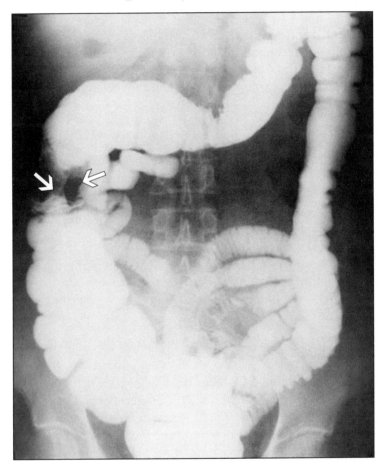

The radiologist may have difficulty identifying a foreign body in the stomach, as opposed to foreign bodies in other structures such as the small intestine or the colon.

• CT scanning may prove more effective than plain X-rays for pinpointing the location of a foreign body and in identifying complications such as perforation and abscess formation.

Foreign body

This upright abdominal plain film of a 14-year-old boy reveals a thumb tack ➜ in the fluid-filled stomach.

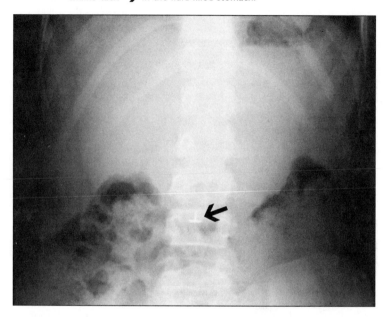

• CT scans may allow the radiologist to view foreign bodies not visible on plain X-rays. Some objects, however, may be seen only after the administration of barium.

⇨ Treatment

Treatment for foreign bodies in the GI tract vary with the type of object and its location. If the object is food, a topical proteolytic enzyme may be ingested to help dissolve the food, depending on its consistency. Extracting the foreign body with a urinary catheter, a snare, a magnetic retrieval device, or another type of suction catheter may be attempted. Endoscopy may be required to remove an object. Surgery is required when foreign bodies cause an intestinal obstruction or when perforation occurs.

Percutaneous gastrostomy tube

The 11-year-old girl on whom this abdominal film was done has cerebral palsy and poor nutrition. The image was obtained after placement of a percutaneous gastrostomy tube. Note the balloon retention device of the gastrostomy tube in the stomach ➡. You can also see the nasogastric tube ➤.

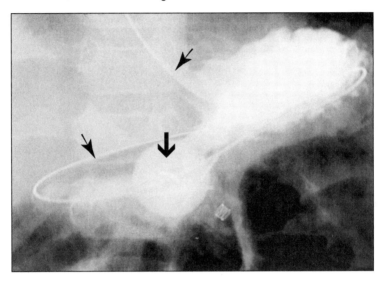

Feeding tubes

Percutaneous gastrostomy, gastrojejunostomy, and jejunostomy feeding tubes are used for functional and mechanical upper GI problems. Indications for placement of a feeding tube include strictures; dysphagia; reflux with aspiration; failure to thrive syndrome; neurologic disorders; oral, pharyngeal, or esophageal tumors; and in cases when long-term, enteral feeding is necessary for the patient's recovery.

Once the diagnosis of poor nutritional status or failure to thrive has been documented, a feeding tube is inserted percutaneously in a radiologic, endoscopic, or surgical procedure. Gastrostomy tubes exit the stomach through an abdominal incision and are held in place by an internal retention device, such as a balloon, a bumper, or a mushroom-type or T-type device. (See *Percutaneous gastrostomy tube.*)

Gastrojejunostomy tubes are inserted into the stomach through the pylorus, just past Treitz's ligament. The tube has a radiopaque band that helps confirm its position. A jejunostomy tube may be placed surgically or radiographically and is inserted directly into the jejunum.

Case study: Small bowel obstruction

A. Barrow, M.D., is a 78-year-old, former family physician with a long history of GI disorders. He suffers from chronic obstructive pulmonary disease (COPD), peptic ulcer disease, and severe esophageal reflux, and he recently suffered a bout of small-bowel obstruction. Forty years earlier, Dr. Barrow had undergone a partial gastrectomy for severe peptic ulcers that didn't heal. After the operation, he developed severe reflux esophagitis with dysphagia and experienced recurrent episodes of aspiration pneumonia, which led to pulmonary fibrosis and COPD. These GI and pulmonary conditions combined to cause Dr. Barrow to become malnourished. His doctor decided he needed enteral feedings to maintain adequate nutrition. Because of Dr. Barrow's history of partial gastrectomy and reflux, his doctor chose to implant a jejunal tube. After tube placement and just before some scheduled diagnostic imaging tests, Dr. Barrow experienced increasing abdominal discomfort. His doctor found that Dr. Barrow's abdomen was distended and that he had tympanitic bowel sounds. Abdominal X-rays revealed a high-grade obstruction of the small bowel.

A small-bowel follow-through subsequently pinpointed the precise site of the obstruction. (See *Small-bowel follow-through examination*, page 164.)

Dr. Barrow was treated conservatively, receiving I.V. fluids to replace lost fluids, an NG tube to decompress his bowel, famotidine I.V. to decrease gastric acidity, methylprednisolone sodium succinate to treat his pulmonary complications, and morphine sulfate to control his pain. Follow-up abdominal

Small-bowel follow-through examination

Dr. Barrow's follow-up study, done by injecting contrast medium through his nasogastric tube, shows a dilated contrast-filled small bowel ⇒. The contrast did not progress past the site of the obstruction.

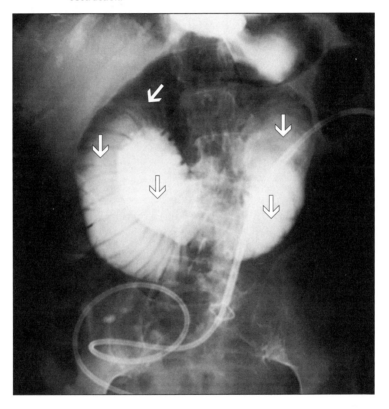

X-rays showed a slight lessening of abdominal gas but no significant relief of the obstruction. Dr. Barrow was scheduled for surgery the next morning. During surgery, doctors found constricting adhesions. The surgeon freed the adhesions and inserted several jejunal stents. Doctors were greatly concerned about Dr. Barrow's poor nutritional state. A jejunostomy tube couldn't be used after surgery, so Dr. Barrow's doctor instituted TPN through an implanted chest port. On the fourth post-

Fecal impaction

This supine abdominal X-ray shows a fecal impaction in the right colon ➜. Note the jejunal tube.

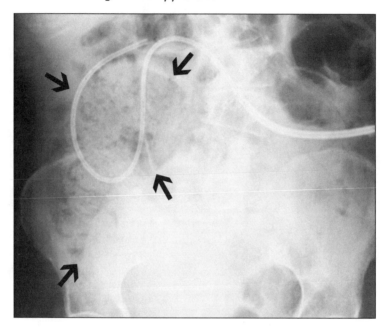

operative day, Dr. Barrow's ileus resolved and tube feedings were restarted. Bowel activity proved inadequate, however. Dr. Barrow frequently aspirated food he was given and as a result, pulmonary complications set in. Doctors stopped his tube feedings and instituted an aggressive pulmonary-treatment regimen. After 4 days, Dr. Barrow's lungs improved, but he had not yet had a bowel movement.

Results from an abdominal series were encouraging. The X-Rays revealed no obstruction, though a significant amount of stool was seen in the right colon. (See *Fecal impaction.*) A gentle, single-dose enema restored bowel activity. Tube feedings resumed, and TPN was gradually tapered off. Twenty days after his arrival at the hospital, Dr. Barrow went home to the care of his wife and a visiting nurse.

Guide to patient care

This chart lists patient preparation and pretest and posttest care for various diagnc imaging tests of the GI system.

Test	Pretest care
Barium swallow	• Restrict food or fluids after midnight the night before the test. • Withhold antacids, as ordered. • Have the patient put on a hospital gown without metal snaps and remove jewelry, dentures, hair clips, and other objects that might obscure anatomic detail in the X-ray films.
Upper GI series and small bowel series	• Instruct the patient to maintain a low residue diet for 2 to 3 days before the test. • Restrict food and smoking after midnight the night before the test. • As prescribed, withhold oral medications after midnight. Anticholinergics and narcotics should be withheld for 24 hours before the test. • Antacids may also be withheld for several hours before the test. • Have the patient put on a hospital gown without metal snaps and remove jewelry, dentures, hair clips, and other objects that might obscure anatomic detail in the X-ray films.

Posttest care	Patient instruction
• Check that additional films are not needed before allowing the patient to resume his usual diet. • Administer a cathartic if ordered. • Inform the patient that his stools will be chalky and light colored for 24 to 48 hours. • Notify the doctor if the patient hasn't expelled the barium within 2 to 3 days.	• Explain that this test evaluates the function of the pharynx and esophagus. • Describe the milkshake consistency and the chalky taste of the barium preparation. • Explain to the patient that he will be instructed to drink about 12 to 14 oz of fluid during the test.
• Be sure no further X-rays are ordered before allowing the patient to resume his usual diet and take oral medications. • Administer cathartics as ordered. • Record and describe all stools. • Notify the doctor if the patient hasn't expelled the barium within 2 to 3 days.	• Explain that this procedure examines the esophagus, stomach, and small intestine through X-ray films taken after the ingestion of barium. • Explain that the procedure may take up to 6 hours to complete. Encourage the patient to bring reading materials with him. • Inform the patient that he'll be placed on an X-ray table that rotates into vertical, semivertical, and horizontal positions. • Describe the milkshake consistency and chalky taste of the barium mixture. • Inform patient that he may be instructed to drink up to 20 oz of fluid. • Inform the patient that his stools will be light colored for 24 to 72 hours.

Test	Pretest care
Barium enema	• Administer a bowel prep as ordered. Enemas may be ordered until the returns are clear. • Restrict dairy products and allow a liquid diet for 24 hours before the test. • Encourage the patient to drink water or other clear liquid for 12 to 24 hours before the test to ensure adequate hydration. • Withhold breakfast if the test is scheduled for the morning. If the test is schedule for the afternoon, give a clear-liquid breakfast.
Colonoscopy	• Restrict diet to clear liquids for 48 hours before the test. • Administer a laxative (such as 10 oz of magnesium citrate or 3 T of castor oil) in the evening, as ordered. Administer a warm tap water enema or a sodium biphosphate enema 3 to 4 hours before the test as ordered, until the returns are clear.

Posttest care

Patient instruction

• Make sure further studies haven't been ordered before allowing the patient to resume his usual diet.
• Encourage extra fluid intake, as ordered, to replace lost fluids. The bowel prep and the test itself can cause dehydration.
• Administer a mild cathartic or a cleansing enema as ordered.
• Record and describe all stools.

• Explain that this test examines the large intestine through X-ray films taken after a barium enema.
• Inform the patient that he may experience cramping pains or the urge to defecate as the barium or air is introduced.
• Instruct patient to breathe deeply and slowly through his mouth to ease discomfort.
• Tell patient to keep his anal sphincter tightly contracted against the rectal tube.
• Inform the patient of the importance of retaining the barium in order to adequately coat the intestinal walls.

• Monitor the patient's vital signs until stable.
• After sedation has worn off, resume the patient's usual diet.

• Explain that this test examines the lining of the large intestine.
• Explain that the test requires a flexible instrument to be passed through his anus.
• Inform the patient that he may receive a sedative, I.M. or I.V., to help him relax.
• Assure the patient that the colonoscope is well lubricated, that it initially feels cool, and that he may feel the urge to defecate as the tube is inserted and advanced.
• Instruct the patient to breathe deeply and slowly through his mouth to relax.
• Explain that air may be introduced into the large intestine through the colonoscope. The air distends the intestinal wall, providing a better view of the lining. Explain also that the patient cannot control the flatus that will escape around the tube.
• Tell the patient to expect a large amount of flatus after the test as air used to distend the colon escapes.
• Inform the patient that he may find blood in his stool if a polyp was removed.

Test	Pretest care
Plain X-ray films of the abdomen	• No food or fluid restrictions are required. • Have the patient put on a hospital gown without metal snaps and remove jewelry and other objects that might obscure anatomic detail in the X-ray films.
Esophagogastroduodenoscopy	• Restrict food and fluids for 6 to 12 hours before the test. • Administer pretest sedation as ordered. • Have the patient remove dentures, eyeglasses, necklaces, hairpins, combs, and constricting garments.

Posttest care

- No posttest care is required.

Patient instruction

- Explain that this test reveals the size and shape of the structures of the abdomen.
- Ensure that the female patient isn't pregnant.

- Observe the patient for possible perforation. Perforation in the cervical area of the esophagus produces pain on swallowing and with neck movement. Thoracic perforation causes substernal or epigastric pain that increases with breathing or with movement of the trunk. Diaphragmatic perforation produces shoulder pain and dyspnea. Gastric perforation causes back or abdominal pain, cyanosis, fever, or pleural effusion.
- Monitor vital signs every 15 minutes for 4 hours, then every hour for 4 hours, then every 4 hours for 24 hours.
- Withhold food and fluids until the patient's gag reflex returns.
- Provide symptomatic treatment of sore throat.

- Explain that this test permits visual examination of the lining of the esophagus, the stomach, and the upper duodenum.
- Inform the patient that a flexible instrument will be passed through his mouth.
- Explain that if the test is done in an emergency situation, the doctor will aspirate stomach contents through a nasogastric tube.
- Tell the patient that a blood sample may be drawn prior to the procedure.
- Inform the patient that a local anesthetic may be sprayed into his mouth to inhibit the gag reflex. Explain that the tongue and throat may feel swollen.
- Explain that a mouth guard will be inserted to protect the patient's teeth and the endoscope.
- Instruct the patient to let saliva drain from the side of his mouth.
- Inform the patient that he'll receive a sedative before the endoscope is inserted but that he will remain conscious.
- After the procedure, instruct the patient to immediately report persistent difficulty in swallowing, pain, fever, black stools, or bloody vomit.

Selected references

Dettenmeir, P.A. *Radiographic Assessment for Nurses.* St. Louis: Mosby–Year Book, Inc., 1995.

Diseases. Springhouse, Pa.: Springhouse Corp., 1993.

Eisenberg, R.L. *Gastrointestinal Radiology,* 3rd ed. Philadelphia: Lippincott-Raven Publishers, 1995.

Gore, R.M., et al. *Textbook of Gastrointestinal Radiology,* vol. 2. Philadelphia: W.B. Saunders Co., 1994.

Laudicina, P. *Applied Pathology for Radiographers.* Philadelphia: W.B. Saunders Co., 1989.

Illustrated Manual of Nursing Practice. Springhouse, Pa.: Springhouse Corp., 1994.

Lewis, S.M., and Collier, I.C. *Medical-Surgical Nursing: Assessment and Management of Clinical Problems,* 4th ed. St. Louis: Mosby–Year Book, Inc., 1995.

Marieb, E.N. *Human Anatomy and Physiology,* 3rd ed. Redwood City, Ca.: Benjamin/Cummings Publishing Co., Inc., 1995.

McCance, K.L., and Huether, S.E. *Pathophysiology: The Biological Basis for Disease in Adults and Children,* 2nd ed. St. Louis: Mosby–Year Book, Inc., 1994.

Taveras, J.M., and Ferrucci, J.T. *Radiology: Diagnosis-Imaging-Intervention,* vol. 4. Philadelphia: J.B. Lippincott Co., 1996.

5 Hepatobiliary system

The hepatobiliary system consists of the accessory glands and organs of the gastrointestinal system. These glands and organs include the liver, gallbladder, pancreas, and the biliary duct system.

Anatomy

The glands and organs of the hepatobiliary system perform many crucial functions. The liver itself plays many regulatory and metabolic roles and is one of the body's most important organs. For digestion, the liver produces bile (a fat emulsifier) to be used by the duodenum. In its metabolic role, the liver processes nutrient-laden venous blood received from digestive organs. The gallbladder's principal role is to store bile. The pancreas, another important component of the hepatobiliary system, produces digestive enzymes released into the small intestine and hormones released into the blood stream.

Liver

The liver typically weighs about 1.4 kg. Located under the diaphragm, the liver extends farther to the right of the body's midline than to the left. The liver has four lobes: the large left and right lobes, and the smaller caudate and quadrate lobes. The caudate lobe is located behind the right lobe; the quadrate lobe, below the left lobe. A delicate mesentery cord, the falciform ligament separates the left and right lobes and suspends the liver from the diaphragm and anterior abdominal wall. A peritoneal extension called the lesser omentum anchors the liver to the lesser curvature of the stomach. The hepatic artery and portal vein, both of which enter the liver, and the common bile duct, which leaves the liver, all travel through the lesser omentum to reach their destinations.

The gallbladder, which stores bile, lies in a recess on the underside of the liver's right lobe. Bile leaves the liver through several ducts that eventually fuse to form the hepatic duct. The hepatic duct joins the cystic duct, which drains bile from the gallbladder, to form the common bile duct.

The liver is composed of units called lobules. Each lobule is a hexagonal, roughly cylindrical structure of plates formed by hepatocytes, or epithelial parenchymal cells. Hepatocyte plates radiate from a central hepatic vein running vertically through each lobule. At each of the six corners of a lobule is a triad region (portal tract), so named because three structures are present there: a branch of the hepatic artery (functional blood supply of the liver); a branch of the portal vein (carrying venous blood from the digestive viscera); and a bile duct. Blood-filled spaces called sinusoids lie between hepatocyte plates. Blood coming from the portal vein and the hepatic artery travels through these sinusoids and empties into the central vein.

Hepatocytes have several major functions:

• They produce bile.

• They pick up nutrients from blood that passes through the sinusoids, and they process those nutrients in various ways, such as by storing glucose as glycogen for later use and by using amino acids to make plasma proteins.

• They store the fat-soluble vitamins A, D, E, and K.

• They play an important role in detoxification.

• As a result of hepatocytic activity, blood that leaves the liver through the hepatic veins contains fewer nutrients and waste materials than does blood that enters the liver through the portal vein.

The blood supply serving the liver feeds off the celiac artery, the first large branch of the abdominal aorta. The celiac artery divides into three branches: the common hepatic, the splenic, and the left gastric arteries. The common hepatic artery runs superiorly, branching to the stomach, and then to the duodenum and pancreas before splitting — as the proper hepatic artery— into the right and left hepatic arteries. As the splenic artery passes deep into the stomach, it sends branches

Biliary tract anatomy

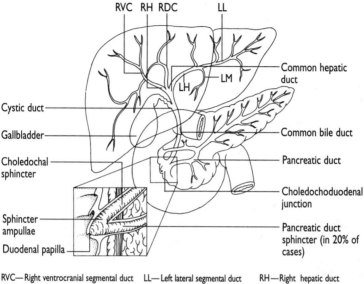

RVC—Right ventrocranial segmental duct   LL—Left lateral segmental duct   RH—Right hepatic duct
RDC—Right dorsocaudal segmental duct   LM—Left medial segmental duct   LH—Left hepatic duct

to the pancreas and stomach and terminates in branches to the spleen. The superior mesenteric artery is a large vessel rising from the abdominal aorta directly below the celiac artery. It runs deep into the pancreas and then enters the mesentery.

Hepatic veins carry venous blood from the liver to the inferior vena cava. Veins draining the digestive viscera form the portal vein, a common vessel that transports venous blood to the liver, where it circulates in the sinusoids before entering the major systemic circulation by way of the hepatic veins. The portal vein supplies about 75% of the liver's blood supply. The hepatic artery supplies the remaining 25%.

Hepatocytes make bile continuously, producing about 500 to 1,000 ml/day. Bile production is enhanced by the secretion of intestinal hormones and bile salts into the blood. Once produced, bile flows through tiny canals, called bile canaliculi, that run between adjacent hepatocytes toward the bile duct branches in the triads. Blood and bile flow in opposite directions in liver lobules. Bile entering the bile ducts leaves the liver by way of the hepatic duct on its way to the duodenum. (See *Biliary tract anatomy,* page 175.) When digestion is not occurring, bile released by the liver makes its way back up the cystic duct into the gallbladder, where it's stored until it's needed.

Gallbladder

The gallbladder is a thin-walled, green, muscular sac about 10 cm long, nestled in a shallow fossa on the ventral surface of the liver. The gallbladder, like most of the liver, is covered by the visceral peritoneum and is served by the same circulatory system that serves the liver. The gallbladder's major function is storing and concentrating bile secreted by the liver. When the muscular wall of the gallbladder contracts, bile is expelled into the cystic duct and flows into the common bile duct.

Although the liver secretes bile continuously, the sphincter of Oddi — which guards the entry of bile and pancreatic juices into the duodenum—is closed when bile is not needed

Gallbladder and cystic duct anatomy

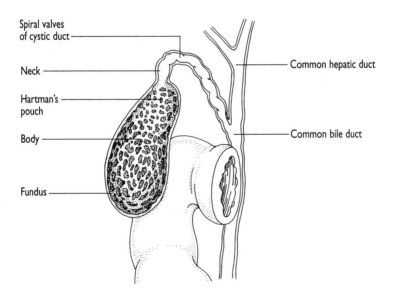

Spiral valves of cystic duct

Neck

Hartman's pouch

Body

Fundus

Common hepatic duct

Common bile duct

for digestion. When that occurs, bile backs up into the gall-bladder and becomes concentrated when the gallbladder's mucosa absorbs water and ions from it. In some cases, the bile released from the gallbladder is 10 times as concentrated as the bile that entered it. (See *Gallbladder and cystic duct anatomy.*)

Pancreas

The pancreas, a soft, pink, triangular gland extending across the abdomen, is the principal enzyme-producing organ of the digestive system. The pancreatic tail abuts the spleen; the pancreatic head is closer to the duodenum. (See *Pancreas anatomy.*) The body and tail of the pancreas are retroperitoneal and lie behind the greater curvature of the stomach.

The exocrine-secretory units of the pancreas, called acini, are clusters of secretory cells surrounding the ducts. Those cells secrete pancreatic juice, an alkaline fluid containing enzymes. Acini are drained by ducts that drain into the centrally located pancreatic duct which, in most people, fuses with the common bile duct just before it enters the duodenum.

Pancreas anatomy

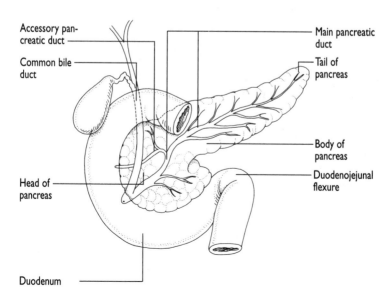

Accessory pancreatic duct

Common bile duct

Head of pancreas

Duodenum

Main pancreatic duct

Tail of pancreas

Body of pancreas

Duodenojejunal flexure

The pancreas also has an endocrine function: It produces two important hormones, insulin and glucagon, that regulate carbohydrate metabolism. Scattered throughout the acinar tissue are the islets of Langerhans, which contain hormone-producing cells.

The pancreas receives blood through the celiac trunk, as do the liver and the gallbladder. The common hepatic artery and the splenic artery serve the pancreas. The superior mesenteric artery runs deep into the pancreas. The splenic vein collects blood from the spleen and from parts of the stomach and pancreas before joining the superior mesenteric vein and forming the portal vein.

Imaging techniques

The following ionizing and nonradiation-dependent technologies provide health care workers with a way of viewing structures within the hepatobiliary system.

Computed tomography

Computed tomography (CT) scanning is considered the workhorse of liver imaging. Iodinated contrast dye to enhance visualization may be injected I.V. or by intra-arterial injection. A CT scan can detect the presence of liver lesions, biliary-system abnormalities, dilated bile ducts, thickened gallbladder walls, and stones. CT scanning also makes it possible to examine structures adjacent to the liver and is the procedure of choice for creating images of the pancreas.

Ultrasonography

Ultrasonography is the preferred method for examining the gallbladder for disease. This imaging technique is excellent for showing stones but doesn't provide information about function or cystic-duct patency. The common hepatic duct is readily seen and can be assessed for obstruction or dilation.

Ultrasonography of the liver is often performed to assess size, fatty infiltration, presence of ascites or lesions, nodularity, vascular anatomy, biliary tree dilation, and other abnormalities.

Although less reliable than CT scanning, it provides excellent images of the pancreas in many patients. Obesity or bowel gas may compromise the quality of the test images.

Oral cholecystography

This technique was considered the standard for diagnosing gallstones until the 1970s when ultrasonography replaced it (except for situations in which cystic-duct patency or the presence of multiple stones needs to be determined). Fat-soluble, oral-contrast tablets (usually six) are taken with a fatty meal 16 to 18 hours prior to filming. The gallbladder is then viewed using plain X-rays.

Nuclear medicine

The Hida scan (technetium-labeled iminodiacetic acid Tc 99m Hida) is a simple procedure for evaluating hepatobiliary function. Morphologic changes of the liver can be observed within 10 minutes after Tc 99m Hida injection. The common bile duct is usually evident within 12 minutes, and the gallbladder typically appears in about 30 minutes. If the gallbladder doesn't appear, suspect acute cholecystitis. The ability to assess function and to obtain morphologic information make Hida scans a valuable tool in hepatobiliary imaging. (See *Normal hepatobiliary scan*, page 180.)

Interventional radiology

Percutaneous transhepatic cholangiography (PTC) offers direct visualization of the biliary-duct system. A fine needle is inserted percutaneously into the bile ducts, and a contrast dye is injected while so-called spot films are taken. Further manipulations within the biliary system can be accomplished by using a combination of guide wires and catheters. Biliary drainage and stent placement may be performed during PTC if obstructions are present.

Hepatic angiography

Hepatic angiography is performed to assess the vascular anatomy of the liver. The radiologist inserts an arterial catheter and

Normal hepatobiliary scan

These Hida-scan images, obtained every 5 minutes after I.V. injection of the isotope TC-99M inert, choletec, show normal liver absorption. Frames 1-3 show normal liver tissue absorbing the isotope. In frame 4, the isotope is in the bile ducts. In frames 5-8, you can see the isotope accumulating in the gallbladder as bile would. Normally, bile's next destination as it passes from the gallbladder is the duodenum. Frames 9 and 10 show the isotope passing from the gallbladder into the duodenum.

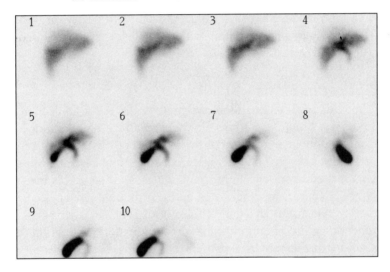

injects contrast dye into the hepatic artery while a series of films is taken. The films help doctors assess arterial blood supply. Delaying filming during the venous phase can demonstrate portal venous structures. Hepatic tumors can be managed with chemoembolization.

Endoscopy

Endoscopic retrograde cholangiopancreatography (ERCP) uses fiber-optic endoscopy, fluoroscopy, and spot filming to assess biliary and pancreatic disease. The gastroenterologist inserts the endoscope into the descending duodenum and locates the papilla of Vater. The pancreatic duct and common bile duct are then entered, using a small plastic catheter.

Contrast dye is then injected and spot films are taken. Less invasive imaging methods — ultrasonography, CT scanning, magnetic resonance imaging (MRI), and nuclear medicine — have replaced many ERCP diagnostic functions, but other therapeutic ERCP applications have been developed, including sphincterotomy, calculi removal, and stent placement. (See *Guide to patient care*, pages 222 to 231.)

Pathophysiology

Like other body systems, the hepatobiliary system is subject to a variety of disorders. Inflammatory and obstructive disorders, tumors, and stones can cause many problems. A large selection of diagnostic and treatment options is available to eliminate or alleviate symptoms of these disorders.

Inflammatory conditions

A host of inflammatory problems, from infection to injury, can plague various components of the hepatobiliary system.

Hepatitis

Hepatitis is a general term for acute or chronic inflammation of the liver. Hepatitis may be caused by viral, bacterial, fungal, or rickettsial infections. Inflammation may follow inhalation, ingestion, or parenteral administration of a number of agents, including alcohol, acetaminophen, halothane, and other drugs.

Viral hepatitis type A (infectious) is transmitted by way of the fecal-oral route and may occur sporadically or epidemically. Its incubation period ranges from 15 to 50 days. The infection usually follows a benign course that doesn't cause chronic hepatitis. Viral hepatitis type B (serum or blood-borne) is transmitted by way of infected blood or body fluids as well as perinatally. The patient may be an asymptomatic carrier or may experience:

* acute hepatitis
* chronic hepatitis
* cirrhosis
* fulminant hepatitis with massive cellular necrosis
* hepatocellular carcinoma.

Viral hepatitis C is caused by a ribonucleic virus transmitted parenterally by blood donors. Usually, this form of hepatitis is transmitted through transfused blood from asymptomatic donors. Symptoms may not occur for as long as 22 weeks after infection. Hepatitis C may cause acute or chronic hepatitis, with 50% of acute cases progressing to chronic.

Type D, also called delta hepatitis, is responsible for about 50% of fulminant hepatitis, which has an extremely high mortality rate. In the United States, type D is confined to people frequently exposed to blood and blood products, such as health care professionals who work with I.V. drug users and hemophiliacs.

Type E hepatitis, formerly grouped with type C as non-A and non-B hepatitis, occurs primarily among patients recently returned from an endemic area, such as India, Africa, Asia, and Central America. It's more common in young adults and more severe in pregnant women.

Alcoholic hepatitis manifests itself as three distinct but overlapping processes: fatty liver, acute hepatitis, and cirrhosis. In most cases, abstinence from alcohol and adequate nutrition may improve symptoms.

⇨ Clinical signs

Symptoms of viral hepatitis include fatigue, anorexia, nausea, vomiting, malaise, mild fever, myalgia, photophobia, pharyngitis, cough, and nasal discharge. Jaundice usually appears 1 to 2 weeks after onset of general symptoms. Hepatomegaly and tenderness occur in 70% of cases. Complete recovery usually takes 3 to 4 months.

Chronic hepatitis is said to occur if inflammatory changes last for longer than 6 months. Prognosis in such cases is usually poor.

⇨ Radiographic findings

The diagnosis of hepatitis usually comes after a clinical workup including the history of symptoms, identification of serologic markers, and confirmation of liver function-test abnormalities. Imaging studies are usually performed to ensure that no obstructive or focal abnormalities exist along with the inflammation. Hepatic-vascular patency may also be assessed.

Ultrasound findings reveal an enlarged liver and spleen.

• A centrilobular pattern is observed in up to 60% of patients with acute hepatitis. This pattern is seen as an increased production or absorption of echoes around the portal veins and a decreased attenuation of liver hepatocytes.

• Mural thickening of the gallbladder may be seen in hepatitis patients.

• The major role of ultrasonography is to exclude biliary obstruction as the cause of liver disease.

CT scanning is useful primarily to exclude focal masses or a hepatocellular carcinoma.

• Findings in hepatitis are often nonspecific although hepatomegaly, gallbladder-wall thickening, and hepatic-periportal lucency are significant signs.

• In advanced disease, ascites, varices, and abnormal liver texture and contours indicate cirrhotic changes.

Nuclear medicine hepatobiliary imaging performed after I.V. injection of a contrast dye can show:

• decreased liver uptake of the tracer

• decreased tracer secretion into the bile ducts and intestine.

⟿ Treatment

There is no effective cure for acute viral hepatitis. Supportive measures, such as rest and a low-fat, high-carbohydrate diet, may help if bile flow is restricted. Administering immune globulin prior to exposure or early in the incubation period can prevent hepatitis A and B.

Cirrhosis

Cirrhosis is a chronic, irreversible inflammatory disease that disrupts liver structure and function. The disease is characterized by parenchymal necrosis and formation of connective tissue that eventually becomes fibrotic. Regeneration of liver cells with nodular tissue results in disorganization of the portal triad (bile duct, portal venule, and arteriole). The liver takes on a knobby appearance and may shrink or enlarge, depending on the stage of the disease.

In early stages of cirrhosis, the liver may swell. In late stages, it may scar and shrink. End-stage cirrhosis is often complicated by portal hypertension and variceal bleeding and by liver failure with encephalopathy and ascites.

Patients with cirrhosis caused by hepatitis or excessive alcohol consumption have a greater than normal risk of developing hepatocellular carcinoma.

➭ Clinical signs

Symptoms appear as the disease progresses from inflammation to hepatic failure. They include fever, pain, nausea, vomiting, anorexia, and fatigue. Signs of liver failure include jaundice, decreased bile in the GI tract (which causes light-colored stools), decreased vitamin K (which causes bleeding tendencies), increased urobilinogen level, dark urine, ascites, and edema. Portal hypertension can lead to variceal formation and hemorrhage. If left untreated, portal hypertension leads ultimately to hepatic encephalopathy, coma, and death.

➭ Radiographic findings

CT scanning is the primary imaging modality for evaluating cirrhosis.
- Fatty infiltration, the initial sign of alcoholic cirrhosis, is typically seen.
- Liver density is less than that of the spleen and hepatomegaly is also evident.
- Later, overall liver volume is diminished.
- Nodularity of the liver contour, fibrous scarring, lobar atrophy, and hypertrophy can be seen with ascites.
- The most characteristic finding on a CT scan is a change

in the caudate lobe–right lobe ratio. The right lobe and the medial segment of the left lobe shrink whereas the caudate lobe and lateral left lobe enlarge. If the ratio exceeds 0.65, a diagnosis of cirrhosis can be made with 96% accuracy.
• CT scanning is also important in screening for hepatocellular carcinoma. (See *Liver cirrhosis*, page 186.)
Ultrasound findings reveal:
• a nodular hepatic contour
• prominence of fissures and porta hepatis
• increased parenchymal echogenicity
• decreased beam penetration
• poor depiction of intrahepatic vessels
• altered gallbladder angle.

➮ Treatment

Removal of toxins, such as alcohol, slows the progression of liver damage and aids liver regeneration. Supportive therapy includes adequate nutrition, administration of vitamin K and lactulose, paracentesis for the removal of fluid, and a low-protein diet to decrease encephalopathy. Control of portal hypertension and subsequent GI bleeding are important aspects of treatment. Portocaval shunting may be performed for intractable ascites or GI hemorrhage that fails to respond to conventional therapy. (See "Treatment," page 203.)

Cholecystitis

Cholecystitis, or inflammation of the gallbladder, is most often associated with cholelithiasis (gallstones). Impaction of a stone in the cystic duct can cause obstruction and inflammation. Eventual bile infection may lead to gallbladder empyema.

Cholecystitis may be acute or chronic. Patients usually report a history of biliary symptoms. These symptoms may include intolerance of fats and cruciferous vegetables, along with heartburn, epigastric discomfort, and flatulence. Acute exacerbation of symptoms is commonly referred to as a gallbladder attack.

Acalculous cholecystitis is rare but may cause severe out-

Liver cirrhosis

In this CT scan, an injected contrast medium shows the liver of a 50-year-old man suffering from the effects of alcoholism. Note ascites ⇒. Also, take note of the gray areas that indicate fibrosis ⇢ caused by cirrhosis scarring in this nonuniformly shaped liver. You can also see the normal stomach **ST** and spleen **SP** on this scan.

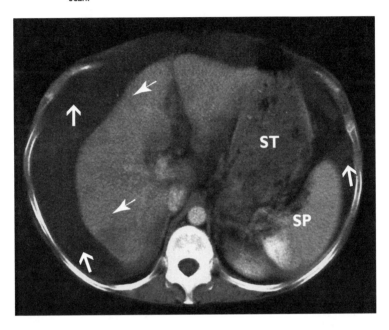

comes. The condition, usually seen in bedridden or debilitated patients, may lead to gangrenous necrosis. It's common in patients with acquired immunodeficiency syndrome.

⇨ Clinical signs

A combination of symptoms — severe right upper quadrant pain, fever, chills, abdominal tenderness, nausea, and vomiting — indicates acute cholecystitis. The white blood cell (WBC) count may be elevated. Liver-function tests and amylase levels may be abnormal. Less acute findings may indicate chronic cholecystitis. Biliary obstruction may occur but is uncommon. Murphy's sign (the arrest of inspiratory effort when gentle finger pressure applied beneath the right sub-costal arch and below the liver margin causes pain during deep inspiration) is a classic sign of acute cholecystitis.

⇔ Radiographic findings

Ultrasonography is the preferred technique for diagnosing cholescystitis. It may reveal the following:
   • Gallstones and Murphy's sign are most frequently identi-fied. In Murphy's sign, the gallbladder is visualized when the ultrasound transducer is placed directly over the most painful part of the abdomen.
   • Ultrasonography also shows a gallbladder that's thickened to greater than 4 or 5 mm, plus gallbladder-wall sonolucency (high or low echo activity, indicating sound waves bouncing off or penetrating the structure) or a halo surrounding the gallbladder, which represents edema from inflammation.
   A Hida scan is also used to diagnose cholecystitis.
   • In this test, failure of the injected radionuclide to accu-mulate in the gallbladder implies cystic-duct obstruction and cholecystitis.
   • Hida scans obtained early in the vascular phase of chole-cystitis may show increased density around the gallbladder fossa and may indicate hyperemia caused by gallbladder inflammation.

⇔ Treatment

The majority of acute attacks resolve spontaneously with pas-sage of a gallstone. Nonsteroidal anti-inflammatory drugs and antispasmodics may help reduce inflammation. Biliary colic without inflammation decreases in several hours. An attack that lasts longer that 24 hours is associated with acute inflam-mation and is less likely to resolve spontaneously. In those cases, antibiotics are needed to treat infections, and narcotics are used to ease severe pain. Suppurative cholangitis (an infection of the bile duct often associated with cholecystitis) may require percutaneous drainage (cholecystostomy), which can ease acute symptoms and stabilize the patient prior to laparoscopic or surgical cholecystectomy. (See *Cholecystostomy tube.*)

Sclerosing cholangitis

Primary sclerosing cholangitis (PSC) is an idiopathic cholestatic (bile accumulation and retention) liver disease. It affects mostly men under age 45. Up to 70% of PSC patients experience associated ulcerative colitis. PSC is characterized by a diffuse inflammatory fibrosis of the biliary tree. The condition may progress to biliary cirrhosis.

Secondary sclerosing cholangitis results from bacterial contamination of static bile, usually from obstruction. Benign obstructions, such as stones, are more likely to lead to cholangitis than are malignant obstructions.

⇨ Clinical signs

Symptoms of PSC include fatigue, pruritus, jaundice, right upper-quadrant pain, and hepatosplenomegaly. Elevated serum alkaline phosphatase and bilirubin levels are often present. Infectious cholangitis symptoms are fever, chills, pain, and elevated WBC count. About 40% of patients with PSC have gallbladder abnormalities, most commonly gallstones.

⇨ Radiographic findings

Direct cholangiography — radiography of the biliary ducts after contrast medium administration — provides definitive diagnostic findings:
• multiple strictures that range from 1 to 2 mm up to several centimeters
• normal or slightly dilated ductal segments interspersed with strictured areas that appear beaded
• obliteration of peripheral ducts that gives a pruned-tree appearance
• ductal-wall irregularities, nodularity, diverticular out-

Cholecystostomy tube

This cholecystogram was taken of a 38-year-old woman with life-threatening colitis who developed acalculus cholecystitis in the ICU. This image was obtained 3 days after a cholecystostomy tube was placed percutaneously. You can see the tube ➜ in the gallbladder.

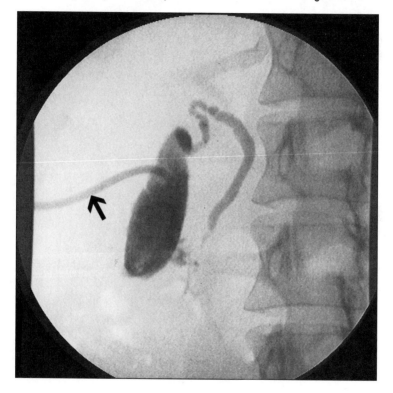

pouchings, and strictures and beading.

ERCP may be performed as well to diagnose PSC. Radiographic appearance will be the same as described above. (See *Primary sclerosing cholangitis*, page 190.)

CT scanning and ultrasonography can show:
- fibrous thickening of the larger bile-duct walls
- cholangiographic signs in less detail
- PSC complications, such as cirrhosis, portal hypertension, and cancer.

Primary sclerosing cholangitis

This image is from a 28-year-old man with ulcerative colitis who presented with jaundice. ERCP shows classic multifocal stricturing of intrahepatic and extrahepatic bile ducts. Note position of the endoscope ➜ and the gallbladder **G**.

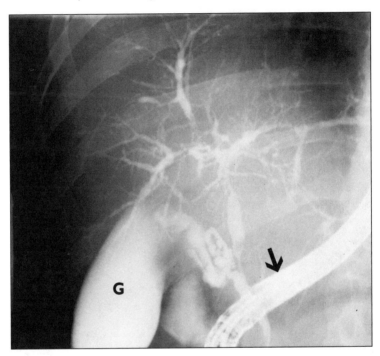

↩ Treatment

Medical therapy for PSC is limited. Prognosis has improved with liver transplantation, but historically, patients with PSC have a median survival rate of 11.9 years from the time of diagnosis. Endoscopic and percutaneous radiologic biliary drainage and stenting have proved useful in treating acute obstruction. Long-term stenting of narrowed bile ducts has had mixed results.

Pancreatitis

Inflammation of the pancreas and peripancreatic tissues is a complex pathophysiologic process. The vast majority of cases of pancreatic inflammation are attributable to either alcoholism or biliary-tract disease (gallstones). Other causes include drug therapy, certain vascular conditions, hyperlipidemia, trauma, anoxia, or infections that activate proteolytic enzymes, leading to autodigestion.

➴ Clinical signs

Symptoms of pancreatitis range from mild abdominal pain, nausea, vomiting, and abdominal distention to severe abdominal pain and shock. Most patients present with abdominal tenderness and guarding. Fever and chills may be present.

Serum amylase and lipase levels and the serum-to-urinary amylase ratio are typically elevated.

Common complications include fluid collections and pseudocyst, phlegmon, and abscess formation. GI hemorrhage, obstruction, ileus, and obstructive jaundice are other complications. Systemic complications such as adult respiratory distress syndrome and shock occur as the disease progresses.

➴ Radiographic findings

In pancreatitis, the goals of imaging studies are to confirm clinical diagnosis of acute pancreatitis, to exclude other abdominal disorders, to evaluate the extent and nature of pancreatic injury, and to assess the condition of adjacent tissue.

CT scanning is the procedure of choice in the diagnosis and management of acute pancreatitis because it shows the entire gland as well as all of its surrounding structures. CT scan findings of pancreatitis include:
- increased pancreatic size
- indistinct margins
- dense accumulation that appears denser than surrounding normal pancreatic tissue
- in advanced disease, intraglandular formation of multiple, small fluid collections

• commonly, pancreatic fluid leaking into the retroperitoneum, usually into the anterior perirenal space
• possible hemorrhagic areas and ascites
• in severe necrotizing pancreatitis, the gland massively enlarged and its edges obliterated by fluid collections dissecting the mesentery and retroperitoneum and possibly extending into the pelvis and up into the mediastinum. (See *Necrotizing hemorrhagic pancreatitis.*)

Factors such as bowel gas limit the usefulness of ultrasonography for assessing patients with acute pancreatitis. It's useful, however, in thin patients with mild edematous pancreatitis and in diagnosing and following the progression of pseudocyst formation.

Plain abdominal X-ray films may be helpful in screening patients believed to have pancreatitis. The most common findings on those films are:
• a duodenal ileus
• a sentinel loop (a dilated, gas-filled segment of small bowel)
• the colon cutoff sign (lack of gas distal to the splenic flexure)
• abscesses characterized by an ill-defined mass associated with a mottled area of gas bubbles in the pancreatic region.

⮂ Treatment

Treatment goals include maintaining stable hemodynamics and fluid volume, relieving pain, and decreasing pancreatic-enzyme production. The patient takes nothing by mouth and has a nasogastric tube inserted to decrease gastric distention and to suppress enzyme secretion. In about 50% of the cases, I.V. fluids and supportive therapy will be required. Also, 40% of patients develop complications that require intervention.

Narcotics can be used to relieve pain. Morphine should be avoided, since it causes spasm of the ampulla of Vater. Histamine-2 blockers are often used to decrease acid production, and antacids are used to neutralize gastric acids. Antibiotics

Necrotizing hemorrhagic pancreatitis

This image is from a 37-year-old female alcoholic suffering from severe necrotizing pancreatitis. A CT scan of the abdomen shows a left upper quadrant mass ⟫ that is denser than normal tissue. The denser material ⟹ is clotted blood in the pancreatic juice forming a hemorrhagic pseudocyst .

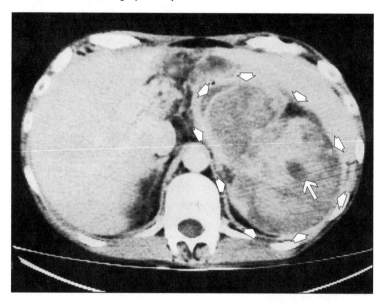

are given to treat underlying infections. Anticholinergic drugs reduce vagal stimulation, decrease GI motility, and stop the production of pancreatic enzymes. Insulin may be needed to treat hyperglycemia.

Surgical or percutaneous intervention may be indicated if biliary obstruction or other complications arise. Sphincter-otomy or biliary stenting using ERCP may help to remove stones or to treat biliary strictures. Percutaneous drainage of pseudocysts or abscesses may also be performed.

Chronic pancreatitis is treated using supportive therapy and by eliminating the underlying cause if possible. Pain relief, replacement of pancreatic enzymes, and insulin therapy may be needed. Surgical intervention may be required to reestablish pancreatic drainage or to alleviate pain. If the patient is debilitated, adequate nutrition should be maintained with hyperalimentation.

Pseudocyst

Pancreatic pseudocysts develop in about half of patients with acute pancreatitis. The fluid in the cyst may consist of pancreatic juices, serum, or blood. The cyst develops from rupture of the pancreatic duct or is secondary to exudation of fluid from the surface of the gland that's caused by activation of enzymes in the pancreas.

The fluid is contained by adjacent structures. Most fluid collections are absorbed within 2 to 3 weeks. Those that aren't reabsorbed encapsulate and form a pseudocyst.

The clinical significance of a pseudocyst is related to its size and potentially lethal complications. Spontaneous rupture into the peritoneal cavity may lead to pancreatic ascites or peritonitis. Abscess formation may occur from secondary infection. Erosion into adjacent blood vessels may lead to massive hemorrhage. Most complications occur when pseudocysts are greater than 5 cm in diameter.

➪ Clinical signs

Symptoms associated with pseudocyst, such as obstruction, pain, and jaundice, arise from displacement and compression of adjacent abdominal organs. Fever and elevated WBC and amylase levels are possible. If the pseudocyst becomes infected, sepsis may occur. Pseudocyst rupture or erosion into a vascular structure may be catastrophic.

➪ Radiographic findings

Pseudocysts vary in size and shape and may be intraglandular or extraglandular.

CT scanning is the best procedure for assessing pseudocyst size and location and may show:
• a low-density fluid collection that's contained by a

Pancreatic pseudocyst

This CT scan shows a mature pseudocyst dense with fluid ▷ in a 29-year-old woman a month after she developed pancreatitis following normal ERCP. Note the pancreatic head ⇒. You can also see the gallbladder **G**, liver **L**, spleen **SP**, and kidneys **K**.

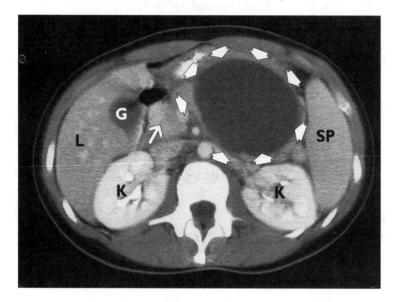

peripheral fibrous capsule and displaces normal structures (see *Pancreatic pseudocyst*)

- gas bubbles that indicate probable infection
- a high-density material that indicates hemorrhage
- pseudocysts that develop outside the pancreas and progress into adjacent or remote structures.

⇨ Treatment

Imaging-guided percutaneous drainage of the pseudocyst is often undertaken in very ill patients. The location of the pancreas, behind the stomach, lends itself to convenient drainage. A large French catheter, #14 to 18, is inserted percutaneously

---

 Pancreatic pseudocyst drainage

These images are from the same woman whose CT scan appears on page 195. Figure A shows a percutaneous drainage tube ⇒, guided by a CT scan, passing through the stomach ➤ and into the pancreatic bed. Fluid has been evacuated. Figure B is an image taken 6 weeks later showing a normal pancreas **P**.

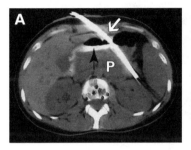 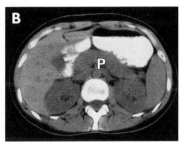

under CT scan guidance through the stomach and into the pseudocyst. A tract forms between the cyst and the stomach within 6 weeks. External drainage is maintained until such a tract forms, at which time the catheter is removed. The tract may allow future accumulations to drain into the stomach and be excreted through the digestive tract. (See *Pancreatic pseudocyst drainage.*)

Some pseudocysts can be drained with an endoscope. If the pancreas is necrotic or hemorrhagic, resection may be the best treatment. Replacement of pancreatic enzymes and hormones may be needed. The patient may also receive antibiotics, analgesics for pain management, and nutritional support.

Obstructions

In a network that has as many ducts as the hepatobiliary system, obstructions are often a problem. As with other body systems, the hepatobiliary system is subject to such blockages as strictures, gallstones, and tumors.

Strictures

Benign strictures of the biliary tree can be caused by a variety of pathologic processes, including trauma, pancreatitis, gallstones, infection, and sclerosing cholangitis. But surgical injury is the most common cause, accounting for 95% of all biliary strictures. Postcholecystectomy strictures are found at the midpoint of the common bile duct near the junction of the cystic duct. If the common bile duct was injured at the time of surgery, more distal strictures can occur.

➭ Clinical signs

Symptoms are related to biliary obstruction. Most commonly seen symptoms include abdominal pain, jaundice, and associated GI tract symptoms, such as nausea, heartburn, clay-colored stools, and dark urine. Elevated serum bilirubin and alkaline phosphatase levels are frequently seen.

➭ Radiographic findings

CT scanning and ultrasonography are used to diagnose biliary obstruction. Ultrasonography may be used first to determine the presence of ductal dilation. CT scanning, however, is usually better than ultrasonography in determining the cause of bile duct obstruction. CT scanning and ultrasonography may show:
- ductal dilation
- stricture without a surrounding mass or stone present.

Cholangiography is used when the results from other non-invasive examinations are normal but when there's a suspicion of obstruction, or when therapeutic interventions are an option. Cholangiography will show:
- benign strictures typically as smooth, focal areas of narrowing and proximal biliary dilation
- a rigid and elongated ampullary segment and delayed common bile duct drainage, which are probable signs of a stricture at the sphincter of Oddi.

ERCP may confirm suspected strictures and diagnose distal obstructions.

⮎ Treatment

Radiographic techniques play an important role in the treatment of benign strictures. Most strictures can be dilated with balloon catheters. Stents are deployed in 80% to 90% of cases. Distal strictures can be treated with ERCP and stent placement, or sphincterotomy can be performed if needed. Yet, even with balloon dilatation and long-term stenting, strictures tend to recur.

Bypass surgery or surgical resection and re-anastomosis can be performed, but these are major surgical procedures that have longer recovery periods than that required for percutaneous or endoscopic treatment. Postoperative scarring may occur as well as a recurrence of stenosis.

Gallstones

More than 25 million Americans have gallstones. Twice as many women as men are afflicted, and the frequency of incidence increases with age. Specific risk factors include obesity, rapid weight loss, ileal disease or resection, hyperalimentation, elevated triglyceride levels, and ethnicity, with members of some Native American tribes more susceptible to gallstones than other people. Most gallstones are made of cholesterol, with bile-pigment stones occurring more frequently in chronic hemolytic disorders.

⮎ Clinical signs

Most people with gallstones are asymptomatic. People who have symptoms usually experience vague or mild ones. The symptom most suggestive of gallstones is 30 minutes or more of postprandial pain in the right upper quadrant. Bloating, nausea, and other GI symptoms may also occur. Once symptoms appear, there's a 50% chance that they'll recur within a year. People who experience frequent gallbladder attacks are at greatest risk of developing acute cholecystitis.

Gallstones

This ultrasonogram is of a 54-year-old woman who complained of pain in her abdomen and back. Note the two low-lying gallstones ⇒ in the gallbladder that are casting a sonic shadow made by the sound waves bouncing off the dense stones. You can see the shadows clearly ⇒.

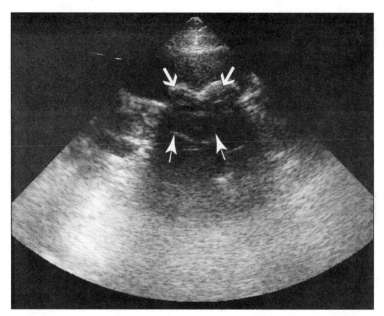

⮌ Radiographic findings

Ultrasonography is by far the best imaging modality for making a diagnosis of gallstones, which are best seen in fasting patients with the gallbladder distended. Ultrasonography will show:

    • a gallstone as an echogenic focus that casts an acoustic shadow and sinks to the bottom of the gallbladder with changes in the patient's position (see *Gallstones*)

    • the tendency of the stone to sink to the bottom of the gallbladder, called gravitational dependence

    • possibly multiple stones that may appear as a layer of

gravel resting on the dependent surface of the gallbladder.

Oral cholecystography is used if ultrasonography is inconclusive or when stones must be counted. It will show:

• a stone as a filling defect in a well-opacified gallbladder, where the structure isn't filled in by contrast dye

• floating stones (usually full of cholesterol) or sinking stones.

Calcified stones may appear on routine abdominal X-ray films as round, opaque objects in the right upper quadrant.

Many stones have the same radiographic density and attenuation as bile, and may not be well differentiated by CT scanning. However, CT scans will show:

• stones with a calcified rim or nidus

• the presence of calcium

• the composition of the stones prior to lithotripsy.

⮞ Treatment

Surgical resection of the gallbladder is one of the most common operations performed in the United States and can be done by laparotomy or by laparoscopy. Several nonsurgical treatments for gallstones are being investigated, including extracorporeal shock-wave lithotripsy, direct-contact dissolution, percutaneous-mechanical extraction, and oral chemolitholysis. Since the advent of laparoscopic techniques, which do not require an abdominal incision, cholecystectomy has become a safer procedure. As a result, interest in alternative techniques has decreased.

Portal hypertension

The portal venous system supplies about 75% of the liver's blood supply. Portal hypertension can be caused by increased total portal venous flow — also known as hyperkinetic portal hypertension — or by increased resistance in the venous system.

Hyperkinetic portal hypertension usually results from a congenital or an acquired arteriovenous (specifically the hepatic artery and portal vein) fistula or shunt. Causes of increased portal-blood flow include trauma to the hepatic or splenic circulation, hepatocellular carcinoma, liver biopsy, transhepatic catheterization, surgery, or rupture of aneurysmal hepatic, splenic, or mesenteric arteries into the adjacent portal-vein circulation.

Resistant portal hypertension can be classified as prehepatic, intrahepatic, or posthepatic.

⇨ Clinical signs

In most cases, patients with portal hypertension have the same signs and symptoms as patients with liver failure. GI hemorrhage caused by esophageal varices is a common problem, as is ascites. Cardiac symptoms similar to those of congestive heart failure may be present, and include edema, labored breathing, and hypertension.

⇨ Radiographic findings

Ultrasonography can help determine the causes of portal hypertension. Findings reveal:
• changes in volume and direction of blood flow in the portal system
• splenomegaly and collateral pathways.
Measuring the portal vein can help diagnose portal hypertension. A portal vein larger than 1.3 cm, for instance, indicates portal hypertension. Other findings include:
• a patent umbilical vein
• splenomegaly with a dilated splenic vein
• ascites and varices
• increased blood flow in the splenic and hepatic arteries and veins.

Color Doppler ultrasonography can detect portal-vein patency and the direction and velocity of portal blood flow.

CT scanning can demonstrate:
• varices
• abnormalities of hepatic size and configuration (nodular appearance)

Esophageal varices

This portal venogram was obtained via the transhepatic route. The image shows esophageal varies in a 38-year-old man with cirrhosis of the liver. You can see the portal vein **P**, the splenic vein **S**, the superior mesenteric vein **SM**, the large coronary vein **C**, and the esophageal varices ➔.

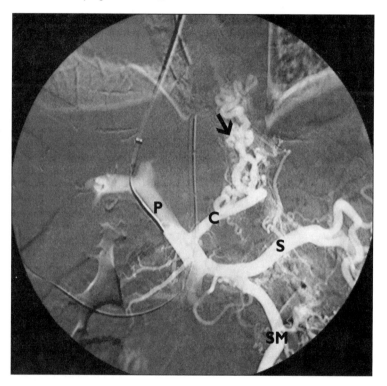

- splenomegaly
- ascites
- portal-vein patency
- invasion or occlusion of the portal venous system by hepatic or other abdominal neoplasms.

Angiography can demonstrate many causes of portal hypertension, including:

- cirrhosis (see *Esophageal varices*)

- tumor
- arteriovenous (specifically the hepatic artery and portal vein) fistula
  - arteriovenous malformations
  - extrahepatic obstruction of the portal vein.

⮕ Treatment

Hemorrhaging esophageal varices can be treated several ways. Endoscopic sclerotherapy can be performed through direct injection of a sclerosing agent into each varix. Vasopressin infusions can decrease portal pressure and temporarily stop acute bleeding. Propranolol can decrease recurrent variceal hemorrhage.

Also, surgical shunt formation may be performed in a variety of ways. Total shunts, such as portacaval, central splenorenal, or mesocaval, or selective shunts, such as distal splenorenal, may decrease portal pressures. Placement of a transjugular intrahepatic portocaval systemic shunt (TIPS) is widely used to treat variceal bleeding and intractable ascites and is particularly useful as a short-term measure prior to liver transplantation.

TIPS is usually performed in an angiography suite by interventional radiologists. The patient is usually sedated with I.V. medications, and a local anesthetic is used at the access point. General anesthesia may be used in patients in whom local anesthesia would be difficult or contraindicated.

Broad-spectrum antibiotics are usually administered prior to the procedure. The radiologist usually places a sheath introducer into the right internal jugular vein. Then, the hepatic vein is catheterized. Special needle sets are used to create a tract from the hepatic vein to the portal vein. The transhepatic tract is then dilated with a balloon catheter. A metal stent is deployed across the tract and dilated from 8 to 12 mm, depending on the patient's pressure measurements. The procedure ends if the portosystemic gradient reaches about 10 mm Hg, and if there is residual portal perfusion and no filling of esophageal varices. Patients are followed periodically with

Esophageal varices after TIPS

This is a portal venogram taken after placement of a transjugular intrahepatic portocaval systemic shunt (TIPS). Note blood flowing through the portal vein **P**. You can also see the hepatic vein shunt → and the emoblic coils ➤ occluding the coronary vein varices to stop them from bleeding.

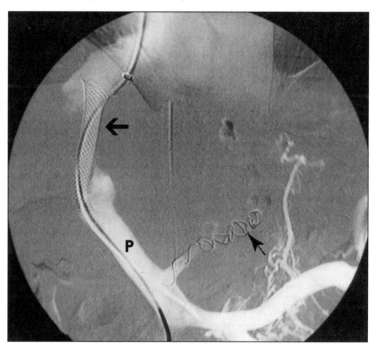

Doppler ultrasonography and venography to ensure patency of the shunt. (See *Esophageal varices after TIPS.*)

Hepatobiliary tumors

Benign and malignant tumors can arise in the hepatobiliary system.

Liver tumors

Malignant tumors of the liver may be primary, arising from hepatic cells, or secondary, arising from lesions elsewhere in the body. Hepatocellular carcinoma (HCC) is the most common malignant primary liver tumor. Predisposing factors for development of HCC include cirrhosis, hepatitis B, and exposure to carcinogens. HCC is one of the most common visceral malignant tumors worldwide and occurs more frequently in men and in patients over age 60.

HCC tumors appear in three distinct growth patterns. Information about those patterns help differentiate tumor type and determine prognosis. Single, or massive, HCC is characterized by a solitary, often large mass. Nodular, or multifocal, HCC presents with numerous well-separated nodules throughout the liver, mimicking the appearance of metastasis. Diffuse, or cirrhotomimetic, HCC is characterized by multiple, small foci located throughout the liver. HCC always occurs as a soft tumor and frequently becomes necrotic and bleeds because of the lack of stroma, or tissue framework. Vascular invasion is common, but biliary invasion is uncommon.

Metastatic disease is the most common cause of malignant liver tumors in the United States. Common primary sites from which metastatic disease arises include the GI tract, breast, lung, and pancreas. Almost half of the people who die from cancer that didn't originate in the liver have liver metastasis.

Cholangiocarcinoma, a malignant tumor that originates in the bile epithelium, is less common than HCC or metastatic disease. Predisposing factors include sclerosing cholangitis, choledochal cyst, familial polyposis, congenital hepatic fibrosis, and toxic exposure to carcinogens. Cholangiocarcinoma may originate from within the liver or outside of it. Four groups of intrahepatic cholangiocarcinoma have been identified according to origin site. They are peripheral, hilar, major hepatic duct, and intraductal papillary cholangiocarcinoma. On imaging studies, these types of cholangiocarcinoma appear as nonspecific mass lesions. Extrahepatic lesions may cause obstruction of the major bile ducts, usually at the confluence of the right and left bile ducts, and at the proximal common hepatic duct. Klatskin tumors are extrahepatic lesions that occur at the bifurcation of the common bile duct. Cholangiocarcinomas of the distal common hepatic or common bile

Bile duct cancer

A 54-year-old woman presented with jaundice and abdominal pain. ERCP shows two sites of bile duct cancer (cholangiocarcinoma), which present as strictures at the confluence of the left and right ducts, a condition that is also known as a Klatskin tumor ⟹. Cancer is also evident in the common bile duct ⟶. The large structure at the bottom of the image is the endoscope ⟹.

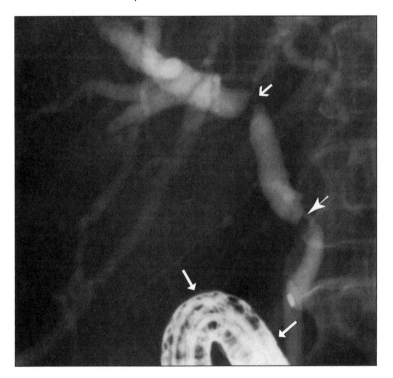

duct are usually small and have a more favorable prognosis than Klatskin tumors because they're easier to resect. (See *Bile duct cancer.*)

Hemangioma is the most common type of benign hepatic tumor. It is five times more common in women than in men. A hemangioma is composed of multiple vascular channels lined by a single layer of endothelial cells. Hemangiomas occur most often in the right lobe and are usually asymptomatic, rarely leading to bleeding. If no symptoms occur, treatment is unnecessary.

⇨ Clinical signs

Symptoms of HCC are insidious at first and include malaise, fever, and abdominal pain. Jaundice is rare. Liver-function tests may be normal. The alpha-fetoprotein level is usually elevated. Most HCC patients in the United States have a long history of alcoholic cirrhosis, hemochromatosis, or steroid use.

Metastatic lesions produce hepatic symptoms in 50% of patients. The most common symptom is hepatomegaly, followed by ascites, jaundice, and varices.

Patients with cholangiocarcinomas usually exhibit jaundice from bile-duct obstruction. Anorexia, weight loss, vague GI symptoms, indistinct upper-abdominal discomfort, and elevated bilirubin and serum alkaline phosphatase levels are also present.

⇨ Radiographic findings

Radiographic findings vary with the characteristics of the tumor.

In HCC, ultrasonography may show:
• variable echogenicity
• diffuse architectural abnormality
• tumor thrombus, with careful analysis of the hepatic and portal veins
• diffuse infiltrating tumors, though possibly difficult to detect.

Metastic involvement of the liver may appear on ultrasonography as:
• fewer echoes (hypoechoic) or more echoes (hyperechoic) than would be produced by a normal liver
• a complex
• a cystlike form.

Hematoma of the liver

This CT scan of the liver was taken of a 51-year-old woman with chronic hepatitis who presented with abdominal pain and weight loss. The scan shows a low-density mass ▶ and central necrosis ⇒. It also reveals enhanced vascularity ⇢ replacing most of the right hepatic lobe. Note the normal left lobe **LL** for comparison, and the spleen **SP** and stomach **ST**.

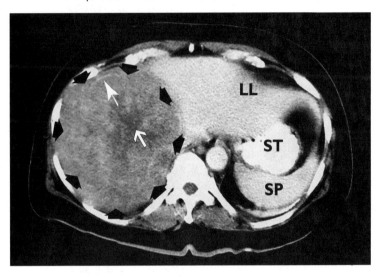

In cholangiocarcinoma, ultrasonography can reveal the extent of bile-duct obstruction but may fail to show tumor mass in as many as 75% of patients.

CT scanning of HCC will show:

• focal HCC as a low-attentuation mass enhanced by a contrast dye injection

• tumor thrombus possibly as a filling defect in the portal or hepatic veins. (See *Hematoma of the liver.*)

Rapid imaging of the liver during administration of an I.V. bolus of contrast dye—a technique known as dynamic sequential bolus CT—is the recommended screening method for metastasis. With metastasis, this technique may reveal:

• low-density lesions (see *CT scan of liver metastases*)

CT scan of liver metastases

This abdominal CT scan is of a 61-year-old man who has colon cancer. Note numerous liver metastases, which appear on the scan as low-density lesions ⇒.

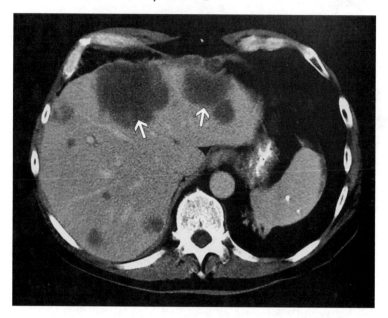

• central areas of markedly decreased density corresponding to central necrosis. (See *CT views of hepatic hemangioma,* page 211.)

In cholangiocarcinoma, CT scanning is more sensitive to obstructive ductal masses, which are usually not as dense as liver tissue.

On MRI, hepatic hemangiomas may display:
• a characteristic response to changes in imaging sequences
• ovoid or spheroid tumors with well-defined edges and no evidence of edema or tissue capsule.

In hepatic hemangiomas, nuclear medicine technetium Tc 99m scans may reveal:
• a classic pattern of a perfusion-blood pool mismatch

• decreased activity early in the scan, then increased activity or delayed images.

Angiographic findings in hepatic hemangioma include:

• a puddling of contrast material in the cavernous vascular spaces.

⤳ Treatment

Resection of the tumor is the treatment of choice for non-metastatic disease. Hepatic chemoembolization is a possible palliative treatment. Radiation therapy may help to shrink tumors and to ease obstruction. Biliary drainage or stenting with percutaneous radiologic technique, or the use of ERCP on obstructed bile ducts may relieve jaundice and associated symptoms. Unfortunately, for most cases of malignant hepatobiliary and pancreatic cancers, treatment is palliative, not curative.

Gallbladder tumors

Gallbladder cancer, the fifth most-common GI-tract cancer, occurs 75% more often in women than in men, and usually between ages 70 and 80. Predisposing factors include cholelithiasis and a calcified, or so-called porcelain, gallbladder. Most gallbladder cancers are adenocarcinomas; the rest are squamous cell carcinomas. Cancer of the gallbladder tends to start in the body of the organ and progress so rapidly that the disease is usually fatal within a year of diagnosis.

⤳ Clinical signs

Most patients with cancer of the gallbladder are asymptomatic in the early stages. Symptoms that appear are usually caused by cholecystitis or cholelithiasis. Later on, severe symptoms may appear when the cancer has spread beyond the gallbladder. Those symptoms include obstructive jaundice, anorexia, weight loss, fatigue, and right upper-quadrant pain.

CT views of hepatic hemangioma

These images were taken of the upper abdomen of a 45-year-old woman who complained of abdominal pain. Figure A, taken before injection of I.V. contrast medium, shows a large, low-density mass in the posterior right lobe of the liver ▷. Figure B, taken during rapid I.V. infusion of contrast medium, shows brightly enhanced vascularity at the periphery of the mass ➔ that is typical of hemangiomas. In figure C, taken 30 minutes after I.V. contrast-medium infusion, the mass is barely perceptible ▶ because it has filled in with contrast medium and become *isodense*, or of the same density as the normal liver tissue.

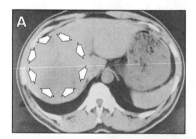

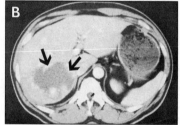

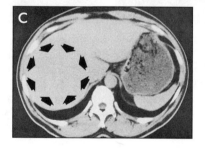

↩ Radiographic findings

Ultrasonography, CT scanning, and MRI are the primary imaging methods for diagnosing cancer of the gallbladder. With both methods, three major patterns appear on cross-sectional imaging:

• focal or diffuse thickening of the gallbladder wall

• polypoid mass originating in the gallbladder wall and protruding into the lumen

CT scan of gallbladder cancer

The first image, figure A, is a CT scan of a 72-year-old woman who presented with weight loss and chronic right upper-quadrant pain. The scan shows a low-density mass ⬠ in the gallbladder fossa extending into the liver. Percutaneous biopsy under the guidance of CT scanning revealed a gallbladder carcinoma. The second image, figure B, is an ultrasonogram of the patient's gallbladder. The image shows an extremely thick gallbladder wall ⇒ with minimal residual lumen ⇢.

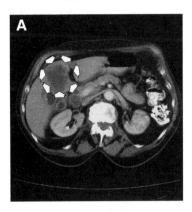

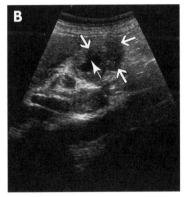

• a mass obscuring or replacing the gallbladder, often invading the liver.

Ultrasonography is limited in its usefulness in diagnosing gallbladder cancer. For instance, calcified stones can block sound waves from the ultrasonography and create a shadow that prevents structures behind the stone from appearing in the image. Calcification of the gallbladder wall may also obscure cancer. Ultrasonography is effective, however, at detecting mural-wall thickening, a nonspecific sign of cancer. The test is also good at revealing polypoid masses in the gallbladder. (See *CT scan of gallbladder cancer*.)

⇨ Treatment

Treatment options for cancer of the gallbladder include surgical removal of the tumor and T-tube drainage and wedge excision of the liver tissues adjacent to the gallbladder. Percutaneous drainage of the common bile duct may relieve symptoms of jaundice and biliary obstruction. Radiation therapy may be palliative; chemotherapy may also be given, although its use is rare. Supportive therapy, such as I.V. infusions, nutrition, and pain-control measures, are important in helping to relieve progressing symptoms.

Pancreatic tumors

Several varieties of tumor can occur in the pancreas. The most common form of pancreatic cancer is duct-cell adenocarcinoma, which accounts for 80% to 90% of malignant pancreatic tumors. Duct-cell adenocarcinoma causes 3% to 7% of all deaths from cancer. Risk factors include cigarette smoking, alcohol consumption, diabetes, chronic pancreatitis, and family history of adenocarcinoma.

⤳ Clinical signs

Cancer of the head of the pancreas causes symptoms such as anorexia, weight loss, pain, fatigue, jaundice, nausea, vomiting, and diabetes. Patients with cancer of the body and the tail of the pancreas are more likely to complain of abdominal pain that radiates to the back. The pain tends to be relieved by bending forward. Those patients are also more likely to experience anorexia and weight loss. In 25% to 50% of patients with cancer of the tail of the pancreas, diabetes may be the sole initial symptom. Venous thrombosis is occasionally found. Physical examination may reveal hepatomegaly, a palpable gallbladder, jaundice, or blood in the stools.

⤳ Radiographic findings

Ultrasonography and CT scanning are useful tools for diagnosing pancreatic cancer.
Ultrasound findings in pancreatic cancer show:
• a focal, hypoechoic (few echoes) mass with irregular margins

CT scans of pancreatic cancer

An 86-year-old man presented with painless jaundice and weight loss. Figure A shows dilated intrahepatic bile ducts ⇒. Figure B shows a distended gallbladder **G** and dilated pancreatic duct ⇒. In figure C, the gallbladder **G**, the dilated pancreatic duct ⇒, and the dilated common bile duct -⊳ are visible. The mass in the pancreas ⇒ is seen in figure D.

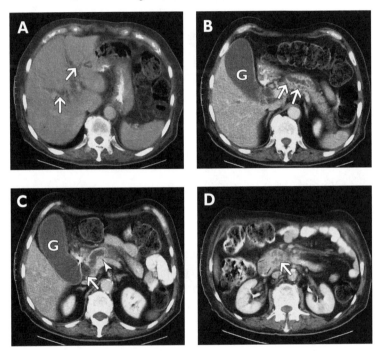

• possible dilation of the pancreatic or bile duct.

Usual CT scan findings include:

• a mass that alters the size and contour of the gland

• a central zone that may be less dense, due to the hypovascular, scirrhous (hard) tumor, whereas the rest of the mass may consist of tissue inflamed by obstructive pancreatitis

• dilation of the main pancreatic duct near the tumor in most cases of cancer of the head of the pancreas and often in cancer of the body of the pancreas

• staging of the cancer, particularly the determination of resectability of the tumor, with lymph-node enlargement and liver metastasis indicating nonresectability. (See *CT scans of pancreatic cancer.*)

PTC is useful in locating strictures or obstructions of the middle or distal common bile duct. PTC also allows drainage if obstruction is present or if guidance for a biopsy is needed.

ERCP is useful in distinguishing masses from focal pancreatitis. Obstruction of the main pancreatic duct is the most common finding.

➪ Treatment

Treatment of pancreatic cancer seldom cures the disease because the tumor tends to metastasize early in its growth. Surgical resection, including partial or total removal of the pancreas, may be performed to try to arrest the spread of cancer. Chemotherapy has shown mixed results in increasing survival time. Combinations of several chemotherapeutic agents may extend life. Radiation may be used to shrink nonresectable tumors and extend life. A number of medications may be required for patients who have had total resections, including insulin, glucagon, enzymes, antacids, anticholinergics, antibiotics, analgesics, and diuretics to relieve ascites.

Catheters, drains, and stents

Various types of catheters, drains, and stents serve many functions in the treatment of hepatobiliary disorders.

Indications

Biliary catheters are indicated for the relief of biliary obstruction and infection or to aid in the dissolution or removal of stones. The main goals of drainage involve ridding the body of accumulated or infectious bile, thereby reducing edema and reestablishing a normal flow of bile. Cholecystostomy is usually done to treat acute cholecystitis or empyema.

Biliary catheters and stents may be inserted percutaneously

T-tube cholangiogram

This T-tube cholangiogram of a 25-year-old woman taken after chole-cystectomy reveals choledocholithiasis with a stone lodged at the ampulla ➔. Note T tube ➤ and the right **R**, left **L**, and common **C** hepatic ducts.

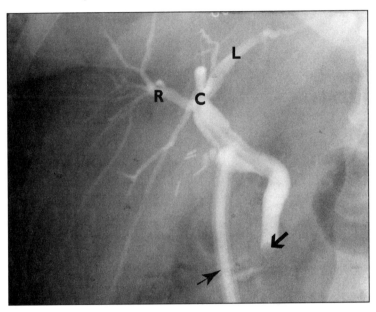

or endoscopically. (See "Case study: A patient's experience with a biliary stent," page 218.) T tubes may be placed during surgery for gallbladder removal if stones remain in the gall-bladder or until the common bile duct heals and normal flow is reestablished. (See *T-tube cholangiogram.*)

Procedure

Percutaneous or endoscopic placement of catheters or stents may be accomplished on a short-stay basis, during which patients remain 6 to 8 hours, or during a 24-hour admission. Prophylactic antibiotics are given and coagulation studies are performed. The patient should have nothing by mouth after midnight and should receive peripheral I.V. fluids.

Percutaneous biliary catheterization

This image is of a 76-year-old woman with metastatic disease obstructing the confluence of the right and left hepatic ducts. The percutaneous catheter ⇒ passes through the right hepatic duct, across the obstruction, and down the common hepatic duct and common bile ducts to the duodenum.

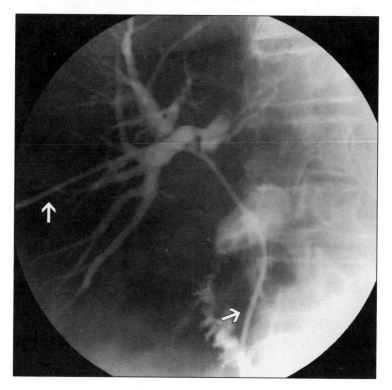

The radiologist gains percutaneous access to the liver with a 22G needle. A midline approach is used for left-lobe access; a right-side approach for the right lobe. A series of catheter and guide-wire manipulations allows the radiologist to insert a #8 or 10 French pigtail catheter into the biliary tree. If the catheter can be inserted beyond the obstruction and into the duodenum, normal flow can be reestablished and internal drainage can occur. For severe obstructions, external drainage may be established by connecting the catheter to a drainage bag.

Depending on the diagnosis and prognosis, an internal stent (endoprosthesis) may be inserted to bridge an obstruction. Stents may be made of plastic or metal. Plastic stents are inserted through a large-bore catheter (#12 French) and have a device on one or both ends for use as an anchor to prevent migration of the stent. The advantage of a plastic stent is that if it becomes occluded, it can be replaced using an endoscope. Metal stents can be inserted through a smaller catheter (#7 French) but cannot be removed once inserted.

Plastic biliary catheters and stents are radiopaque catheters that have a number of side holes for the drainage of bile. The catheter should be placed with holes above and below the obstructing lesion. Most external catheters have a pigtail, or looped, end to help maintain their position in the duodenum.

Injection of contrast dye may be needed to check the catheter's position in the biliary tree. (See *Percutaneous biliary catheterization,* page 217.)

Case study: A patient's experience with a biliary stent

Fifty-four year-old Mrs. Bolinski has a history of gallstones and biliary colic that resulted in a cholecystectomy 20 years ago. She recovered and was relatively free from symptoms.

Two years ago, Mrs. Bolinski was referred to a gastroenterologist because of right upper-quadrant abdominal pain that persisted for 1 month. An ERCP was performed, but the upper biliary tree was not visualized because of a stricture of the middle common bile duct. Mrs. Bolinski was scheduled for a percutaneous cholangiography. If the test revealed biliary obstruction, the radiologist would insert a drain.

The procedure was performed under I.V. sedation. The radiologist found an apparently benign stricture of the proximal common hepatic duct. (See *Stenotic common hepatic duct.*)

Stenotic common hepatic duct

This image is a percutaneous transhepatic cholangiogram using a small catheter ⇒. You can clearly see the severely stenotic common hepatic duct ➤.

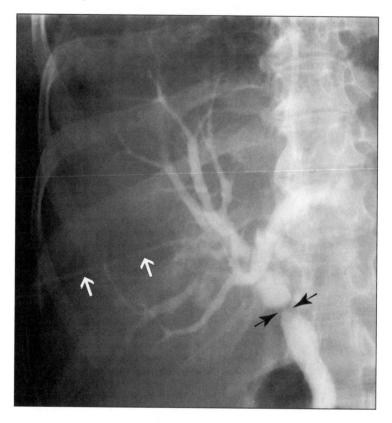

A catheter and guide wire were passed through the stricture and down into the duodenum. A #8.3 French pigtail catheter was then advanced, with some difficulty, across the stricture and was left in place to allow external drainage. After Mrs. Bolinski recovered, she and her husband were informed of possible treatment options. They decided to allow doctors to perform a stricture dilatation and large-stent placement in the hope that the procedure would correct the obstruction. Mrs.

Cholangiogram after stent placement

This test was done after metallic stents ➔ were placed. Note that the contrast dye flows freely through the stents and into the duodenum. No residual stenosis is evident. The internal-external catheter ➔ remains after the procedure as a safety precaution.

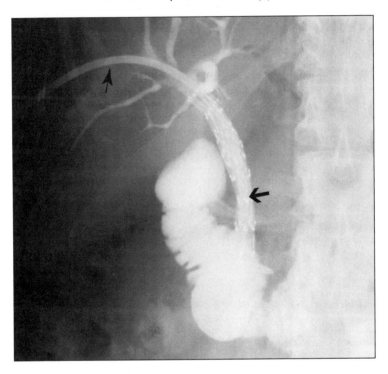

Bolinski requested general anesthesia because of the discomfort she had experienced during the previous procedure.

The next morning, Mrs. Bolinski was given general anesthesia and the biliary catheter was exchanged for a balloon catheter. The stricture was dilatated up to 10 mm, and a #14 French internal-external stent was inserted.

Mrs. Bolinski tolerated the procedure well and left the hospital the next morning. Three weeks later, she experienced some vague abdominal pain, which necessitated a follow-up dilatation. No residual stenosis was seen following contrast dye injection. A #14 French self-retaining biliary catheter was inserted and capped for internal drainage.

Mrs. Bolinski was checked biweekly in the clinic for dressing changes and status reports. After 4 months, she again developed symptoms of biliary colic and abdominal pain. Biliary catheter injection revealed several stones next to the catheter that were partially obstructing the common bile duct. Mrs. Bolinski was readmitted for percutaneous stone removal through the existing tract.

Four stones were removed using a steerable combination catheter and wire basket, and the duct was irrigated. Contrast dye injection revealed that the stricture had recurred. The duct was redilatated to 12 mm, and a #14 French catheter was reinserted.

The next morning, Mrs. Bolinski and her husband were again counseled about treatment options. Because of her history of stone formation and recurring stenosis, and because of the tendency of the biliary tract to become infected easily, Mrs. Bolinski chose to have an internal expandable metal stent inserted. The procedure was scheduled for 1 month later, to allow for postdilatation healing.

Mrs. Bolinski received general anesthesia for the procedure. Three 3-cm Z stents and one 1.5-cm Z stent were passed through the stricture so that the entire hepatic and common bile ducts were stented. No residual stenosis was noted, and rapid flow of contrast dye into the duodenum was accomplished. (See *Cholangiogram after stent placement.*) A #12 French catheter was inserted to maintain access and to allow the closure of the tract.

Mrs. Bolinski was discharged the next morning. A follow-up cholangiogram 10 days later showed that the stent was widely patent and that Mrs. Bolinski was symptom-free. The external drain was downsized to a #8 French catheter.

Two weeks later, Mrs. Bolinski was feeling well and was eager for doctors to remove the external drain. The stent was functioning well without recurrence of stenosis, and the final drain was removed. For the first time in more than a year, Mrs. Bolinski was catheter-free and on the road back to a normal life.

Guide to patient care

This chart lists patient preparation and pretest and posttest care for various diagnostic-imaging tests of the hepatobiliary system.

Test	Pretest care
Liver and biliary tract computed tomography	• Restrict food and fluid after midnight the night before the test if the administration of contrast medium is anticipated. • Note hypersensitivity to contrast medium on the patient's chart.
Liver-spleen scan	• No pretest restrictions on diet are required.

Posttest care	Patient instruction
• Inform patient he may resume his usual diet.	• Explain that this test helps to detect liver and biliary tract disease. • Inform the patient that he will be placed on an adjustable table, he will have to remain still during the test, and he will be asked periodically to hold his breath. • Inform the patient that an I.V. or an oral contrast medium may be given. • Instruct the patient to immediately report nausea, dizziness, sweating, headache, urticaria, or a flushed feeling.
• Observe for signs or symptoms of an allergic reaction. The stabilizer added to the radioactive tracer can cause allergic reactions in sensitive people.	• Explain that this procedure permits examination of the liver and spleen through scans taken after I.V. injection of a radioactive substance. Assure the patient that allergic reactions are rare. • Explain that the detector head of the gamma camera may touch the patient's abdomen. Reassure him that contact with the camera poses no danger to him. • Tell the patient that he will be asked to lie still and to breathe quietly to ensure high-quality images. He may also be asked to hold his breath briefly. • Ensure that the female patient isn't pregnant.

Test	Pretest care
Pancreatic computed tomography	• Restrict food and fluid after midnight the night before the test. • Note hypersensitivity to contrast medium on the patient's chart. • Administer contrast medium, if ordered.
Ultrasonography of the gallbladder and the biliary system	• Restrict diet to a fat-free meal in the evening. The patient then fasts for 8 to 12 hours before the test.
Ultrasonography of the liver	• Restrict food and fluid for 8 to 12 hours before the test to reduce bowel gas.
Ultrasonography of the pancreas	• Restrict food and fluid for 8 to 12 hours before the test to reduce bowel gas. • Restrict smoking just before the procedure.

Posttest care	Patient instruction
• Resume the patient's usual diet.	• Explain that this test is painless and helps to detect disorders of the pancreas. • Explain that the patient will be placed on an adjustable table and will be asked to remain still and, periodically, to hold his breath. • Inform the patient that an I.V. or an oral contrast medium may be given to enhance visualization of the pancreas. Tell him to immediately report nausea, dizziness, sweating, headache, urticaria, or a flushed feeling.
• Make sure to remove all lubricating jelly from the patient's skin. • Resume the patient's usual diet.	• Explain that this procedure allows examination of the gallbladder and the bile-collection system. • Explain that he may feel mild pressure as the transducer passes over the skin. • Instruct him to remain still and to hold his breath when requested, to ensure that the gallbladder is located in the same position for each scan.
• Remove the lubricating jelly from the patient's skin. • Resume the patient's usual diet.	• Explain that this procedure allows examination of the liver. • Assure the patient that the test is painless, but he may feel mild pressure as the transducer is passed over the skin. • Instruct the patient to remain as still as possible during the procedure and to hold his breath when requested.
• Make sure to remove all lubricating jelly from the patient's skin. • Resume the patient's usual diet.	• Explain that this test allows examination of the pancreas. • Assure the patient that the test is not painful but that he may experience mild pressure. • Instruct the patient to inhale deeply when requested and to stay as still as possible during the procedure.

Test	Pretest care
Ultrasonography of the spleen	• Restrict food and fluids for 8 to 12 hours before the test to reduce bowel gas.
Oral cholecystography	• Instruct the patient to eat a meal containing fat at noon the day before the test and a fat-free meal that evening. • Restrict food, fluids (except water), cigarettes, and gum after midnight the night before the procedure. • Administer six tablets (3 G) of iopanoic acid 2 or 3 hours after the evening meal, as ordered. The patient should swallow the tablets one at a time at 5-minute intervals, each pill taken with 2 mouthfuls of water, for a total of 8 oz of water. • Administer a cleansing enema the morning of the test, if prescribed.
Percutaneous transhepatic cholangiography	• Restrict food and fluids for 8 hours before the test. • Administer 1 G of ampicillin I.V. every 4 to 6 hours for 24 hours before the procedure, if prescribed. • Administer a sedative before the procedure, as prescribed. • Note hypersensitivity to contrast medium on the patient's chart.

Posttest care	Patient instruction
• Make sure to remove all lubricating jelly from the patient's skin. • Resume the patient's usual diet.	• Explain that this procedure allows examination of the spleen. • Assure the patient that he will most likely experience only mild pressure during the test. • Instruct the patient to lie as still as possible during the procedure and to hold his breath when requested.
• Resume the patient's usual diet.	• Explain that this test uses X-rays taken after ingestion of a contrast medium to visualize the gallbladder. • Tell the patient to report adverse effects of dye ingestion, including diarrhea (common), nausea, vomiting, abdominal cramps, or dysuria. • Examine emesis or diarrhea for undigested tablets. If present, notify the X-ray department.
• Ensure that the patient rests quietly for at least 6 hours — preferably lying on his right side — to help prevent hemorrhage. • Monitor vital signs until stable. • Check injection site for bleeding, swelling and tenderness. Watch for signs of peritonitis, such as chills, temperature of 102° to 103° F, and abdominal pain, tenderness or distention. • Resume the patient's usual diet.	• Explain that this test uses X-rays taken after ingestion of a contrast medium to visualize the liver. • Inform the patient that he will be placed on a special X-ray table that rotates vertically and horizontally. • Advise the patient that injection of the contrast medium may produce a sensation of pressure and epigastric fullness and may cause transient right upper back pain. • Tell the patient to report symptoms of allergy, such as nausea, vomiting, excessive salivation, a flushed feeling, urticaria, or sweating.

Test	Pretest care
Postoperative cholangiography	• Clamp the T tube the day before the procedure, if necessary. • Withhold any meal scheduled just before the test. • Note hypersensitivity to contrast medium on the patient's chart.
Endoscopic retrograde cholangiopancreatography (ERCP)	• Restrict food and fluids after midnight the night before the procedure. • Obtain baseline vital signs. • Have the patient remove all metal objects and constricting undergarments. • Have the patient void before the procedure to help to relieve the discomfort that may follow the procedure.

Posttest care

Patient instruction

• Change the dressing at the puncture site whenever necessary.
• If a T tube is left in place, attach the tube to a drainage system.

• Explain to the patient that this procedure uses X-ray films taken after the injection of a contrast medium to examine the biliary ducts.
• Tell the patient that he may feel a bloating sensation (not pain) in the right upper quadrant as contrast medium is injected.
• Instruct the patient to report nausea, vomiting, excessive salivation, a flushed feeling, urticaria, or sweating.

• Monitor the patient's vital signs every 15 minutes for 4 hours, then every hour for 4 hours, then every 4 hours for 48 hours.
• Monitor for apnea, hypotension, excessive diaphoresis, bradycardia, or laryngospasm during the first 8 hours after the procedure.
• Withhold food and fluids until the patient's gag reflex returns.
• Check for signs of urinary retention during the first 8 hours after the procedure.
• Provide symptomatic treatment of the patient's sore throat.

• Explain that this procedure uses X-ray films taken after the injection of a contrast medium to examine the liver, gallbladder, and pancreas.
• Inform the patient that a local anesthetic may be sprayed into his mouth to inhibit the gag reflex. The spray may make the patient's tongue or throat feel swollen, causing difficulty in swallowing.
• Instruct the patient to let saliva drain from the side of his mouth.
• Inform the patient that a mouth guard will be inserted to protect his teeth and the endoscope.
• Assure the patient that he will receive a sedative before insertion of the endoscope but that he will remain conscious.
• Warn the patient that he may experience transient flushing when the contrast medium is injected. Advise him to report feelings of nausea, vomiting, flushing, urticaria, or sweating.
• Advise the patient that he may have a sore throat 3 to 4 days afterward.
• Inform the patient that he may receive an anticholinergic or glucagon I.V. after insertion of the endoscope. Describe possible adverse effects of anticholinergics (dry mouth, thirst, tachycardia, urinary retention, and blurred vision) and of glucagon (nausea, vomiting, hives, and flushing).

Test	Pretest care
Hida scan	• Restrict food and fluids for 2 hours before the test.
Abdominal radiography	• No food or fluid restrictions are required. • Have the patient put on a hospital gown without metal snaps and remove jewelry and other metal objects that might obscure anatomic detail in the X-ray films.

Posttest care

Patient instruction

• Observe for signs or symptoms of an allergic reaction. The stabilizer added to the radioactive tracer can cause allergic reactions in sensitive people.

• Explain that this procedure uses scans taken after I.V. injection of a radioactive substance to examine the liver, biliary system, gallbladder, and duodenum.
• Assure the patient that allergic reactions to the radioactive substance are rare.
• Explain that the head of the gamma camera may touch his abdomen, but that contact with the camera poses no danger.
• Inform the patient that he will be asked to lie still and to breathe quietly. He may also be asked to hold his breath briefly.
• Ensure that the female patient isn't pregnant.

• No posttest care is required.

• Explain that this test reveals the size and shape of abdominal structures.
• Ensure that the female patient isn't pregnant.

Selected references

Diseases. Springhouse, Pa.: Springhouse Corp., 1993.

Eisenberg, R.L. *Gastrointestinal Radiology,* 3rd ed.
Philadelphia: Lippincott-Raven Publishers, 1996.

Gore, R.M., et al. *Textbook of Gastrointestinal Radiology,* vol. 2.
Philadelphia: W.B. Saunders Co., 1994.

Loeb, S., et al., eds. *Handbook of Medical-Surgical Nursing.*
Springhouse, Pa.: Springhouse Corp., 1994.

Marieb, E.N. *Human Anatomy and Physiology.* Redwood City,
Calif.: Benjamin/Cummings Pub. Co., 1989.

McCance, K.L., and Huether, S.E. *Pathophysiology: The
Biological Basis for Disease in Adults and Children.* St. Louis:
Mosby–Year Book, Inc., 1990.

Taveras, J.M., and Ferrucci, J.T. *Radiology: Diagnosis-Imaging-
Intervention,* vol. 4. Philadelphia: J.B. Lippincott Co., 1994.

6 Genitourinary system

Disorders of the genitourinary system—renal and urologic problems — affect 8 million people in the United States. Chances are good, then, that health care professionals will encounter these patients often.

Anatomy

The genitourinary (GU) tract consists of the kidneys, the ureters, the urinary bladder (which stores urine), and the urethra (which carries urine out of the body). (See *Genitourinary tract anatomy,* page 234.)

The kidneys bear the major responsibility for eliminating toxins, drugs, and nitrogenous wastes from the body. The kidneys also produce the enzyme renin, which helps regulate blood pressure and kidney function, and the hormone erythropoietin, which stimulates red blood cell (RBC) production in bone marrow.

Kidneys

The bean-shaped kidneys lie in the superior lumbar region, between the parietal peritoneum and the dorsal body wall. They extend from the level of about T12 to L3 and are protected by the lower part of the rib cage. The right kidney, crowded by the liver, lies slightly lower than the left. The typical adult kidney weighs about 156 g and is about 11.4 cm long, 7.6 cm wide, and 2.5 cm thick. The lateral surface of the kidney is convex, while the medial surface is concave and has a vertical cleft called the hilus that leads to the renal sinus. Two ureters and a number of renal blood vessels, lymphatic vessels, and nerves enter the kidney at the hilus and occupy an area called the renal sinus. Atop each kidney is an adrenal (suprarenal) gland.

Genitourinary tract anatomy

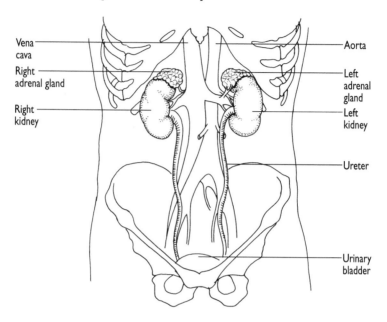

Vena cava
Right adrenal gland
Right kidney
Aorta
Left adrenal gland
Left kidney
Ureter
Urinary bladder

Kidney regions

Three distinct regions form the kidney. The outer region, or cortex, houses the renal tubules and glomeruli, which play roles in fluid filtration and absorption. The middle section, or medulla, contains cone-shaped filtering systems called medullary pyramids (or renal pyramids). The broader base of each pyramid faces the renal cortex; its apex, or papilla, faces the inner region. Urine that passes through the pyramids drains into the calyces — cup-shaped areas that collect urine and empty it into the renal pelvis. Urine then flows into the ureter, which transports it to the bladder for storage. (See *Internal kidney anatomy*, page 236.)

Blood supply

The kidneys have a rich supply of blood and continuously clean it and adjust its composition. Under resting conditions, the renal arteries deliver about one-fourth of the total cardiac output (about 1,200 ml) to the kidneys each minute. The renal arteries arise at right angles from the abdominal aorta between L1 and L2. The left renal artery is typically shorter than the right. Prior to entering the kidney, the renal artery divides into five lobar, or segmental, arteries that enter the kidney at the hilus. Each lobar artery then branches to form several interlobar arteries that pass between the medullary pyramids and into the cortex. The interlobar arteries themselves divide into branches called arcuate arteries, which curve over the bases of the medullary pyramids. Small interlobular arteries run upward from the arcuate arteries to supply the cortical tissue.

More than 90% of the blood entering the kidney perfuses the cortex, which contains the nephrons — the structural and functional units of the kidneys. Blood leaving the renal cortex drains first into the interlobular veins and then into the arcuate veins, the interlobar veins, and the lobar veins before finally draining into the renal veins. Blood in the renal veins empties into the inferior vena cava, which lies to the right of the vertebral column. Because the inferior vena cava is located closer to the right kidney than to the left, the right renal vein is about half as long as the left renal vein.

Ureters

The ureters are slender tubes, each about 28 cm long and 0.6 cm wide, which carry urine from the kidneys to the bladder. A slight bend in the ureter as it enters the bladder prevents backflow of urine when the bladder fills or empties. Urine is propelled through the ureters by peristaltic waves initiated in the renal pelvis. An initial peristaltic wave forces urine from the pelvis into the ureter, distending the ureter with urine. That distention stimulates contraction of the ureter and propels urine into the bladder.

The body adjusts the frequency and the strength of those peristaltic waves according to how quickly urine forms. Peristaltic waves may occur several times a minute or only once every several minutes.

Internal kidney anatomy

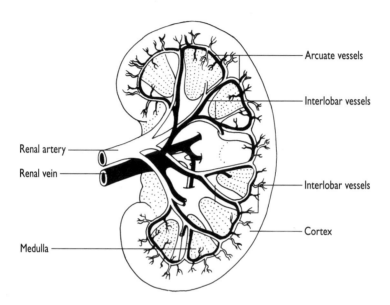

Arcuate vessels

Interlobar vessels

Renal artery

Renal vein

Interlobar vessels

Cortex

Medulla

Bladder

The urinary bladder is a smooth, collapsible muscular sac located retroperitoneally on the pelvic floor just posterior to the symphysis pubis. (See *Bladder and urethra anatomy.*)

In men, the bladder lies immediately in front of the rectum, and the prostate gland surrounds the bladder neck. In women, the bladder lies near the vagina and uterus anteriorly.

The interior of the bladder contains openings for the ureters and for the urethra. The triangular region formed by these three openings is called the *trigone.*

The bladder is quite distensible and uniquely suited for its urine-storing function. When there's little or no urine, the bladder collapses to a length of about 6.4 cm. When urine accumulates, the bladder expands and becomes pear-shaped. A full bladder can distend to about 12.7 cm long and can hold about a 480 ml of urine. In some cases, however, the bladder can hold more than double that amount. When severely distended, the bladder becomes firm and can be palpated well above the symphysis pubis.

Mucus produced by the bladder mucosa helps protect the bladder wall from stagnant urine. That protection is particularly important when the urine is more acidic or more alkaline than normal.

Urethra

The urethra is a thin-walled muscular tube that drains urine from the bladder out of the body. A thickening of the smooth muscle at the bladder-urethral junction forms the internal urethral sphincter, which is an involuntary sphincter that keeps the urethra closed when urine is not being released. A second sphincter, the external urethral sphincter, is controlled voluntarily and is fashioned by skeletal muscles as the urethra passes through the pelvic floor.

Bladder and urethra anatomy

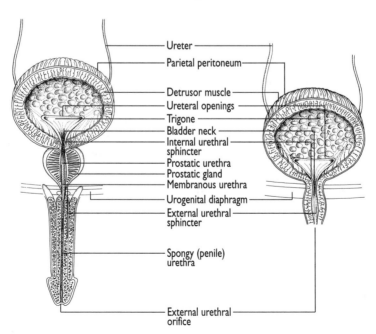

- Ureter
- Parietal peritoneum
- Detrusor muscle
- Ureteral openings
- Trigone
- Bladder neck
- Internal urethral sphincter
- Prostatic urethra
- Prostatic gland
- Membranous urethra
- Urogenital diaphragm
- External urethral sphincter
- Spongy (penile) urethra
- External urethral orifice

In women, the urethra is 3.8 cm long and tightly bound to the anterior vaginal wall by fibrous connective tissue. Its external opening, the external urethral orifice (meatus), lies anterior to the vaginal opening and posterior to the clitoris. In men, the urethra is about 20.3 cm long and has three parts. The prostatic urethra, about 2.5 cm long, is surrounded by the prostate gland. The membranous urethra extends a short distance from the prostate gland to the beginning of the penis. The spongy urethra, or penile urethra, is about 15 cm long. It passes through the penis and opens at its tip through the external urethral orifice. The male urethra carries semen and urine out of the body.

Imaging techniques

Radiologists can use a number of techniques to gain a clear picture of the health of the GU tract.

Ultrasonography

Ultrasonography, or ultrasound, has supplanted excretory urography as the best method for diagnosing subacute or chronic urinary obstruction. Ultrasonography is also valuable for assessing kidney size and for diagnosing renal masses. It can also yield useful information about reflux, diverticula, urine retention, and bladder size. Duplex ultrasonography can confirm blood flow in a kidney's venous or arterial system.

Computed tomography

Computed tomography (CT) scanning is the premier method for diagnosing urinary tract tumors, particularly renal cell carcinoma and renal metastasis. It's also preferred for evaluating kidney trauma and renal calculi.

Excretory urography

Excretory urography (formerly called intravenous pyelography) is performed on patients who may have a urinary tract infection, neoplasm, acute GU pain, hematuria, neurogenic bladder, congenital anomalies, or renal and ureteral calculi or who have experienced trauma. The test is also performed on patients who have had or will have renal transplantation or who are suffering from certain postoperative complications. A kidney-ureter-bladder (KUB) film is taken prior to injection of a contrast dye. The KUB can detect abnormalities such as calculi, which may be obscured by the dye.

In excretory urography, an I.V. contrast dye is administered, and X-rays are taken at timed intervals. A compression band — a constricting plastic waistband that compresses the patient's abdomen to help distend the upper urinary tract — is applied to help distend the upper urinary tract. The patient may also be put in a supine position.

The patient often receives bowel preparation the evening before the examination to help prevent bowel gas from interfering with the test. The patient should be well hydrated the day of the examination to allow for faster excretion of the contrast dye and to prevent renal toxicity and dehydration from the dye.

Voiding cystourethrography

Voiding cystourethrography (VCUG) is performed to check for abnormalities of the bladder and urethra and to determine the status of vesicoureteral reflux. VCUG is performed by inserting a catheter into the bladder and instilling a contrast dye until a sufficient amount of fluid has distended the bladder to full capacity. After the catheter is removed, the patient is asked to void. Fluoroscopy is then used to detect any reflux of urine into the ureters.

Interventional radiology

Interventional radiology, which includes antegrade pyelography and retrograde pyelography, deals with diagnosis and treatment of GU disorders. These and other tests are useful for a number of procedures, including percutaneous nephrostomy catheter placement, percutaneous calculi removal, internal ureteral stenting, needle biopsy, and renal cyst aspiration.

Retrograde pyelography

A retrograde pyelography study is performed by inserting an endoscope through the urethra and into the bladder. The ureter is then cannulated and injected with contrast dye for viewing the ureter and collecting system.

Antegrade pyelography

Antegrade pyelography is used to diagnose kidney and ureteral conditions when retrograde access is not possible. An antegrade pyelogram is performed by percutaneous placement of a needle or catheter in the renal collecting system and injection of contrast dye for viewing the collecting system and ureter.

Nuclear medicine

Nuclear medicine tests, in which various radioactive materials are used to see organs or other structures, can provide information about renal blood flow, nephron function, and urinary drainage. Such tests are relatively simple and expose the patient to minimal discomfort and low levels of radiation.

Vesicoureteral reflux may be evaluated by instilling a radionuclide into the bladder and scanning for ureteral filling. Urinary obstruction can also be detected by these tests. The drug furosemide may be administered I.V. during a renogram to enhance the diagnosis of partial obstructions.

Magnetic resonance imaging

Magnetic resonance imaging (MRI) is often used to assess the GU system. The test is especially helpful in patients who can't tolerate iodinated contrast dye. MRI can detect a renal mass but may be unable to determine whether the mass is solid or cystic. MRI also isn't very effective for detecting calcifications.

MRI angiography, use of magnetic resonance imaging along with a contrast dye, can be used to test for renal artery stenosis, to assess vascular malformations, and to design a preoperative plan. (See *Guide to patient care*, pages 272 to 279.)

Pathophysiology

Like any system of the body, the GU system is subject to disease and other conditions that affect the function of its organs and other structures.

Inflammatory conditions

Inflammatory conditions that affect the GU system include pyelonephritis and cystitis.

Pyelonephritis

Pyelonephritis can be divided into two categories: acute and chronic. Acute pyelonephritis is an infection of the renal pelvis usually caused by bacteria that enter the bladder through the urethra or by blood-borne pathogens. The condition is seen most often in women between ages 15 and 40. The short urethra in women predisposes them to infection. The longer urethra in men, combined with the antibacterial properties of prostatic secretions, helps protect men against such infection.

Infection is often limited to one kidney lobe, with a sharp line of demarcation between inflamed tissue and normal tissue. Inflammatory exudate may fill and obstruct collecting tubules and ducts, which leads to diminished urine formation in the affected nephrons. The whole kidney may be edematous because of an inflammatory response.

The offending organism is most often *Escherichia coli*. Following acute infection, inflammation may resolve without damaging the kidney. Inflammation may also worsen into bacterial nephritis or renal abscess. Fortunately, most patients respond well to antibiotic therapy without more serious complications.

Chronic pyelonephritis is believed to be the end result of vesicoureteral reflux with or without accompanying infection. The resultant anatomic renal abnormalities may be seen long after the reflux has been corrected. The disease causes scarring that can extend from the calices to the surface of the kidney. The affected parenchyma can become atrophic and be replaced by fibrous tissue.

Tubules are usually absent in the scars, and any remaining glomeruli are dilated, atrophic, and filled with an amorphous, sludgy fluid. The papillary region is usually retracted outward and the periphery is retracted inward, which causes the affected calices to become distended and blunted. Occasionally, reflux is severe enough to make the entire kidney hydronephrotic, which thins the parenchyma. Overall kidney size is usually diminished in such cases.

✎ Clinical signs

Acute pyelonephritis
Patients with acute pyelonephritis usually experience a sudden onset of fever, chills, flank pain, urinary frequency, and dysuria. Blood studies often reveal leukocytosis. Urinalysis usually shows bacteria, leukocytes, leukocyte casts, and RBCs.

Chronic pyelonephritis
Most patients with chronic pyelonephritis are young women. The patient may suffer from hypertension, show symptoms of chronic renal failure, or have a history of renal calculi or recurrent urinary tract infections. Urinary frequency, dysuria, and flank pain may also be present. Many patients relate a history of chronic urinary infections throughout childhood. Urinalysis may reveal white blood cells (WBCs) with or without bacteriuria.

✎ Radiographic findings

Acute pyelonephritis
In one of four patients, X-rays can detect acute pyelonephritis within 24 hours of symptom onset. X-ray findings using excretory urography are:
- most commonly, global enlargement of the affected kidney
- occasionally, bilateral global enlargement, even though symptoms are unilateral
- delayed enhancement of renal tissue (delayed or diminished nephrogram)
- delayed filling of the collecting system, which appears as

asymmetric, decreased contrast in the affected collecting system and ureter
• caliceal compression — a displacement or narrowing of the contrast-filled collecting system by the swollen areas of the inflamed kidney. (See *Right pyelonephritis*, page 244.)
A CT scan may reveal the same abnormalities as those found on excretory urography, but the findings are characterized by sharply defined, wedge-shaped zones of diminished contrast. These zones radiate from the collecting system to the renal surface. (See *Left pyelonephritis*, page 245.) CT scanning is also the preferred method for diagnosing renal-abscess formation and may be useful in guiding the placement of a percutaneous drain.
Ultrasonography can indicate acute pyelonephritis by showing:
• smooth, swollen kidneys that have a thickened corticomedullary area that doesn't produce echoes.
However, ultrasonography may not be able to differentiate an early abscess formation from edema.
Nuclear medicine imaging demonstrates:
• the same pattern of multifocal, wedge-shaped areas of diminished renal function as ultrasonography does.

Chronic pyelonephritis
Excretory urography of a patient with chronic pyelonephritis reveals:
• focal scars or regions of thinning parenchyma, with each scar tending to retract the surface of the kidney inward while distending the calyx outward, leading to a clublike appearance of the calyx
• decreased kidney size
• severe scarring, which may lead to hypertrophy of normal portions of the parenchyma.
CT scanning will show:
• scars as focal regions of thinned parenchyma.
Ultrasonography may reveal:
• scarring as an area of parenchymal loss and increased echoes.

Right pyelonephritis

This excretory urogram was taken of a 28-year-old woman who had a fever, right flank pain, and pus in her urine. The pyelogram revealed a swollen right kidney ⬦. Look at how the kidney is swollen, especially the upper pole.

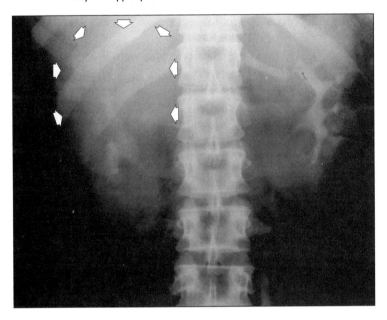

Nuclear medicine scanning will show:
- large areas of damage as an asymmetry of renal function
- diminished size of the affected kidney.

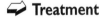 Treatment

Acute pyelonephritis

Acute pyelonephritis is treated with antibiotics. Anti-inflammatory medications may be administered to help decrease edema. Increased fluid intake is encouraged to flush the exudate out of the system. Renal abscess can usually be treated with I.V. antibiotics but may require percutaneous radiographic drainage or surgery. If obstruction is present, per-

Left pyelonephritis

This is a CT scan of a 31-year-old woman who presented with sepsis, a temperature of 103° and a white blood cell count of 18,700. The image shows a swollen left kidney with wedge-shaped areas of diminished enhancement involving the cortical and medullary tissue ➔. The normal right kidney appears uniform ➤.

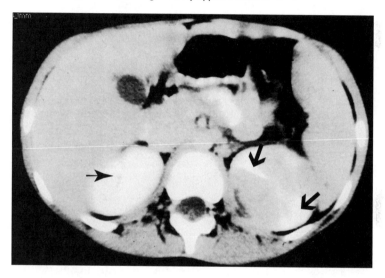

cutaneous nephrostomy is often required to relieve hydronephrosis and to control infection.

Chronic pyelonephritis

Antibiotics are also used for chronic pyelonephritis. Therapy involves treating underlying causes, particularly obstruction. The patient may require antihypertensives or diuretics to treat hypertension. When the patient suffers renal failure, dialysis or kidney transplantation may be necessary.

Cystitis

Cystitis is an acute or chronic condition in which the bladder wall becomes edamatous and inflamed. Hemorrhagic cystitis is a type of cystitis in which small hemorrhages occur in the bladder mucosa.

Cystitis is caused primarily by bacterial infection. Other causes include radiation therapy; medications such as cyclophosphamide; urinary stasis or reflux; obstruction, as with prostatic hyperplasia; and instrumentation after catheterization or cystoscopy. Cystitis is more common in women than in men because women have shorter urethras, and because of the proximity of the urethra to vaginal and anal bacteria.

⇦ Clinical signs

Signs and symptoms of cystitis include dysuria, urinary frequency and urgency, lower pelvic pain, and fever. Cystitis causes the urine to be cloudy and malodorous with pus, bacteria and, often, RBCs.

⇨ Radiographic findings

Cystography — radiography of the bladder after an opaque solution is injected into the organ — may be done if the patient does not have an acute infection. In cystitis, this technique typically reveals:
- a thicker-than-normal bladder mucosa with a cobblestone appearance (caused by mucosal inflammation and edema)
- reduced bladder capacity
- obstructing lesions, which may be the cause of cystitis.

⇨ Treatment

Antibiotic therapy is administered if urine studies determine which bacterium is causing the infection. For some patients, such as women with an uncomplicated acute infection, single-dose antibiotic therapy may be sufficient to clear the infection.

Other patients, such as those with prostatitis, may require longer courses of antibiotics. If cystitis is medication-induced, the drug may be stopped. The patient should drink plenty of fluids. To prevent reinfection, any underlying bladder-outlet obstruction should be relieved.

Congenital disorders

Congenital anatomic variations can lead to significant problems in the GU tract.

Vesicoureteral reflux

Normally, the angle of the ureter entering the bladder forms a kind of one-way valve that prevents the reflux of urine into the ureter. When that angle is insufficient, the valve may open and reflux of urine may occur. Reflux may occur only during voiding, when bladder pressure is high, or at any time. The degree of reflux is divided into diagnostic grades, depending on the results of VCUG, as follows:

• Grade I indicated by opacification of the distal portion of the ureter

• Grade II indicated by opacification of the entire ureter and collecting system without dilation

• Grades III and IV indicated by opacification of the entire urinary tract with varying degrees of dilation of the calyces and intrarenal regions.

Vesicoureteral reflux is most often seen in young girls. As the patient grows older, the length of the submucosal tunnel of the ureter may increase, and the valve mechanism may become competent. A strong correlation exists between urinary tract infection and reflux. Urinary tract infections and certain anatomic abnormalities may predispose some people to reflux. Posterior urethral valves, bladder-outlet obstruction, and neurogenic bladder dysfunction may all be causes. The major concern with long-standing reflux is eventual development of chronic pyelonephritis, which is believed to occur when vesicoureteral reflux is severe and pressure in the renal pelvis is high enough to force fluids from the calices to flow backward into the collecting tubules. Such retrograde flow is referred to as intrarenal reflux and may cause focal renal damage. Intrarenal reflux most often affects the upper poles of the kidney.

⇨ Clinical signs

Young patients with reflux often experience symptoms of urinary tract infection. Many patients remain asymptomatic until renal damage has occurred.

If symptoms are present, they include fever, frequency, dysuria, flank pain, and malaise. Urinalysis can reveal WBCs and bacteriuria in people with concurrent infections.

⇨ Radiographic findings

Fluoroscopic VCUG is the classic imaging technique for demonstrating vesicoureteral reflux. It reveals the following findings:
• reflux prior to or during voiding, after a contrast dye is instilled into the bladder by urinary catheter
• when reflux is present, varying degrees of opacification or dilation of the upper tracts
• most significantly, dilation of the upper urinary tract and intrarenal reflux. (See V*esicoureteral reflux.*)

Excretory urography isn't usually performed to diagnose reflux but may be done in conjunction with VCUG to assess the upper urinary tract. Excretory urography may yield the following findings:
• evidence of chronic pyelonephritis
• dilation of the upper tract
• hydronephrosis.

Radionuclide cystography is frequently used for follow-up examinations after initial VCUG has been performed. Its advantages include:
• detection of vesicoureteral reflux while delivering a lower radiation dose to the patient
• detection of transient reflux that routine tests might miss, because patients are scanned longer during this procedure than during routine radiography.

Vesicoureteral reflux

This is an image of a 3-year-old boy who had recurrent urinary tract infections. A voiding cystourethrogram was performed with contrast dye injected through a catheter placed in the bladder by way of the urethra. You can plainly see the contrast-filled bladder **B**. Massive left-sided reflux up the dilated ureter ➔ and into a dilated collecting system ⇥ is also seen.

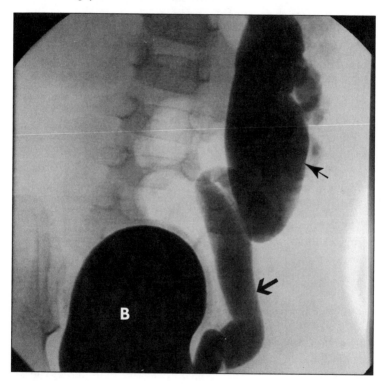

⇦ Treatment

Antibiotics are administered for patients with infections. Long-term maintenance doses may be given to prevent reinfection. In mild cases among young people, the patient is kept infection-free without invasive therapy in the hope that the distal ureter will grow long enough to resolve the problem.

Surgery is often reserved for severe cases of reflux leading to kidney damage. In this procedure, known as ureteroneocystostomy, the distal ureter is removed from the bladder and reimplanted so that the submucosal tunnel is relatively long.

Renal vascular disorders

The GU system is subject to the same types of vascular disorders that affect the rest of the body.

Renovascular hypertension and arteriosclerosis

Renovascular hypertension is systemic hypertension caused by stenotic disease of the major renal arteries. Atherosclerosis, a type of arteriosclerosis, is the most common cause of renal stenosis and accounts for two-thirds of all cases of renovascular hypertension. Stenosis may occur in normotensive or hypertensive patients. Common complications of atherosclerotic plaques include ulceration, thrombus, hemorrhage, calcification, aneurysm, and dissection. High-grade renal stenosis generally leads to total occlusion within a year.

The condition affects mostly people over age 50. The most common site of stenosis is the proximal 2 cm of the renal artery. Lesions typically produce an irregularity of the lumen and sometimes poststenotic dilation.

⇔ Clinical signs

The most common finding in renal arterial disease is hypertension that doesn't respond well to drug treatment. A bruit (a vibration-like sound) may be heard over the abdomen at the level of the renal arteries. In severe cases, renal perfusion may be compromised, leading to decreased urine production in the affected kidney.

⇔ Radiographic findings

Angiography is the primary method for diagnosing renal artery stenosis. Classic angiographic findings include:
  • calcifications in the main renal artery. (See *Renal artery*

Renal artery stenosis and occlusion
This angiogram shows left renal artery stump ➔ and high-grade
right renal artery stenosis ➔> .

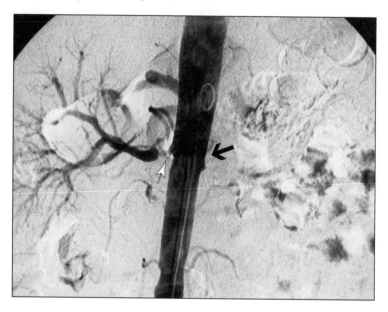

stenosis and occlusion and *Renal artery stenosis corrected by stenting,* page 252.)

Other possible angiographic findings include:
• stenotic dilation
• affected kidney smaller than the nonaffected one.

During angiography, renal vein sampling for renin evaluation may be done as a screening aid to determine if the patient's hypertension is renovascular.

Nuclear medicine studies in renal artery stenosis often reveal:
• asymmetry in the rate of radioactivity, the time taken to reach peak activity, and the decline of activity in each kidney.

Nuclear medicine studies can also be used to determine if more invasive studies are warranted. Using captopril in conjunction with a radionuclide can help diagnose renal artery disease as a cause of hypertension.

Renal artery stenosis corrected by stenting

In the first image, figure A, an aortogram reveals an occluded right renal artery ➜ in a 68-year-old man who presented with hypertension and renal failure. The left renal artery has a high-grade, irregular atherosclerotic stenosis ➤. The second image, figure B, made by renal angiography, shows the left renal artery opened after balloon angioplasty and insertion of a stent. Serum creatinine levels went from 3.8 to 1.6. Hypertension did not improve.

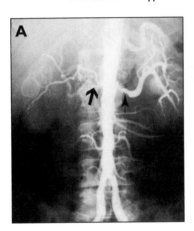

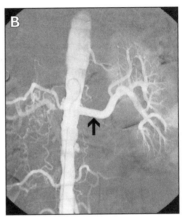

Doppler ultrasound arterial-flow studies are also used as a screening aid. Renal stenosis is indicated by:
- a widening and an elevation of the waveform tracing.

↩ Treatment

Most cases of hypertension are not renovascular in origin and are managed with drugs and diet. When medications are unable to control hypertension, angiography or other tests may be performed to assess status or to plan treatment. Renal artery angioplasty can be performed at the time that the tests are done, if indicated. In severe cases when angioplasty is not possible or when it fails, a surgical bypass or even a nephrectomy may be considered.

Fibromuscular dysplasia

Fibromuscular dysplasia (FMD) consists of a group of lesions with fibrous, muscular, or fibromuscular hyperplasia. The disease process may involve the arterial intima, media, or adventitia. Medial fibroplasia with mural aneurysm is the most common type of FMD and accounts for up to 70% of cases. One-third of renal artery stenoses are caused by FMD. The condition affects women more often than it does men and usually occurs among people ages 30 to 40.

⮩ Clinical signs

Hypertension is the most common sign of FMD, especially hypertension that doesn't respond well to treatment. An abdominal bruit may also be present.

⮩ Radiographic findings

Medial fibroplasia usually affects the distal two-thirds of the main renal artery or its branch vessels. The condition is characterized by alternating areas of aneurysm and stenosis that on a plain X-ray film look like a string of beads, which is diagnostic of the disease.

⮩ Treatment

Balloon angioplasty is highly effective for medial fibroplasia and can avoid long-term antihypertensive therapy.

Obstructions

Urinary tract obstructions may occur in many different locations and for a variety of reasons. An obstruction may be located within the urinary system (called intrinsic) or outside the system (called extrinsic). Causes of intrinsic obstructions include calculi, blood clots, edema from a calculus or an infection, transitional cell carcinoma or other primary urinary tract tumors, and a number of other less common causes. Causes of extrinsic obstructions include pregnancy, pelvic or malignant retroperitoneal disease, benign prostatic hyperplasia, and inflammatory processes of the abdomen, pelvis, or retroperitoneum.

Functional obstructions occur from loss of ureteral peristaltic activity or loss of bladder-muscle function, which occurs with vesicoureteral reflux and neurogenic bladder.

Urine-flow interference can cause stasis and increased hydrostatic pressure. Accumulation of urine above the obstruction can lead to infection or damage of the involved structures, either of which may result in renal failure. Early diagnosis and intervention is essential to prevent permanent damage.

Renal calculi

Calculi form in the kidney as crystalline aggregates with an ordered structure and a sequential growth pattern. Saturation level of a given ion or molecule in the urine can lead to calculus formation.

Factors that influence calculus formation include urinary pH, body temperature, urine volume, and absence of a substance excreted by the kidneys that inhibits formation of crystals (which precede calculi). Urinary stasis and foreign material in the collecting system also favor calculus formation. About 90% of the calculi that occur in people in the United States contain some form of calcium. The other 10% are calcium-free and consist mostly of uric acid or cystine.

Systemic conditions that promote calculus formation include a urine-inhibitor deficiency, dietary hyperuricuria, hypercalciuria, hyperparathyroidism, prolonged immobilization, milk-alkali syndrome, neoplastic disorders, Cushing's syndrome, and urinary tract infections.

Calculi may occur alone or in groups and can be found anywhere in the collecting system. They can cause obstructions when they lodge in narrowed areas, such as the ureteropelvic junction or the distal ureter-bladder junction. Intermittent obstruction can result when calculi move. Hydronephrosis may occur if the ureter is blocked completely. (See *Obstructing ureteral calculus.*)

Obstructing ureteral calculus

This 51-year-old man presented with severe right flank pain. The intravenous pyelogram shows a dilated right renal collecting system ⇒ and proximal ureter. The opaque calculi ⇥ obstructing the ureter are partially hidden by the contrast. The left collecting system ⟹ and ureter ▷ are normal.

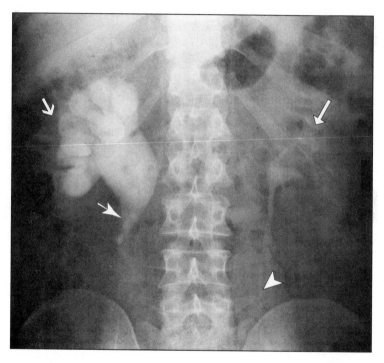

⮎ Clinical signs

Acute symptoms may result from movement of calculi through the urinary system. The patient may experience renal colic, a crescendo-decrescendo pattern of severe flank and abdominal pain that can radiate into the groin, scrotum, or labia. Hematuria is usually present. Symptoms of urinary tract infection, such as fever, painful urination, and dysuria, may also occur.

⟜ Radiographic findings

KUB X-rays and excretory pyelography reveal most renal calculi. Injection of contrast medium further enhances calculi appearance on X-ray films.

The radiographic appearance of a calculus depends on its composition. Some calculi are dense and radiopaque; others have a mixed composition and a radiopaque core. Still others may be entirely radiolucent. Plain X-rays may show the following.

• After a contrast dye mixes with the urine, certain calcium-containing calculi appear as bright white spots, indistinguishable from the pure contrast. Other calculi, those that contain cystine or uric acid, become radiolucent in the presence of dye.

• Calculi may appear round, smooth, or jagged.

• Rapidly growing stones tend to branch and form staghorn shapes. (See *Right renal staghorn calculus.*)

• Kidney ultrasonography reveals strong echoes and an acoustic shadow with a sharp margin when a calculus is present. Ultrasonography is not accurate for diagnosing small intrarenal calculi or ureteral calculi. However, it does detect such obstructing changes as hydronephrosis.

• CT scanning without I.V. contrast dye can demonstrate urinary tract calculi. CT scanning is better than standard radiography because it can differentiate various densities and many calculi that are not detected by standard X-rays.

⟜ Treatment

Calculi are treated according to location and composition. Extracorporeal shock wave lithotripsy (ESWL) uses external sound waves to break calculi into small particles that then pass out of the body in the urine. Percutaneous lithotripsy can be performed through nephrostomy access. A device is inserted through a nephrostomy tube and fragments the calculus directly. This technique is used for large calculi that can't be disrupted by the less invasive ESWL. Lower ureteral or blad-

Right renal staghorn calculus

This plain X-ray film of a 70-year-old woman who hadn't received I.V. contrast shows a branching staghorn calcification ⇛ filling the right renal collecting system.

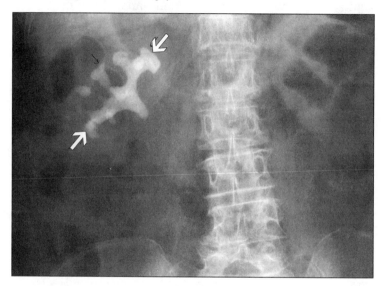

der calculi can be removed using cystoscopy and retrograde calculus extraction. Surgical intervention is usually reserved for large staghorn calculi that can't be removed through other, less invasive means.

Bladder-outlet obstruction

Bladder-outlet obstruction can be mechanical, functional, or neurologic. Causes of mechanical obstruction include tumors, calculi, ureteroceles, urethral strictures, inflammatory disease of the prostate or urethra, tumors of the prostate, and conditions that occlude the external meatus. Causes of functional or neurologic obstruction include neurologic impairment of the detrusor muscle and some central nervous system lesions.

When the bladder is obstructed, the detrusor muscle becomes hypertrophied, which results in trabeculation and thickening of the normally smooth bladder wall. The trigonal region also becomes enlarged. The bladder mucosa herniates and produces cellules, saccules and, eventually, diverticula.

Long-standing obstruction can lead to decreased detrusor contractibility, residual urine retention, and atony of the bladder wall.

Increased intravesical pressure may be transmitted to the upper urinary tract. This may lead to an upper-tract obstruction that affects function, which results in dilation of the ureter and collecting system, leading to renal failure. Cystitis and pyelonephritis can occur as a result of stagnant urine or urinary infection. Stone formation is another complication of bladder-outlet obstruction.

➷ Clinical signs

Common complaints associated with bladder-outlet obstruction include hesitancy in starting a urinary stream, a weak or intermittent stream, postvoid dribbling, urinary frequency, nocturia, and a feeling of incomplete emptying. Upper-tract symptoms, including flank pain and fever, are rare unless infection is present. Nausea, malaise, and weight loss suggestive of uremia may also exist.

➷ Radiographic findings

Plain X-ray films may reveal:
• a distended bladder
• bladder calculi
• prostatic calcifications.

Excretory urography is the diagnostic procedure of choice for evaluating outlet obstruction. It can detect:
• residual urine
• bladder-wall trabeculation
• diverticula
• calculi
• other complications of bladder-neck obstruction.

VCUG under fluoroscopic guidance allows examination of

Vesicoureteral reflux

This voiding cystourethrogram was obtained from a 3-year-old boy with a neurogenic bladder. Note the irregularly shaped bladder **B**, the reflux into the dilated left ureter **U**, and the contrast in the proximal urethra ➔.

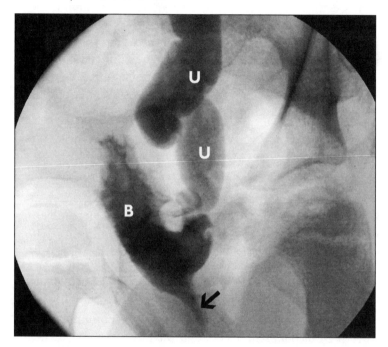

the bladder and urethra. Spot films taken during voiding can demonstrate reflux. (See *Vesicoureteral reflux.*)

CT scans may reveal:

• diffuse thickening of the bladder wall in cases of cystitis or tumor involvement

• bladder calculi (which may be observed without the aid of contrast medium).

Ultrasonography may be used to evaluate the prostate as a possible cause of the bladder-outlet obstruction. Ultrasonography of the upper urinary tract is a highly reliable screening tool for dilation, which may result from reflux or obstruction.

A filled bladder can be evaluated for diverticula, calculi, tumors, and estimation of residual urine volume.

⮑ Treatment

The treatment of choice for bladder-outlet obstruction is the relief of the obstruction. Surgical resection of an enlarged prostate, a tumor mass, or a repair of other urethral abnormalities may be indicated. Medical management of neurologic problems include medications to enhance bladder contractibility, antibiotics to combat infection, and possible intermittent self-catheterization to maintain urinary flow.

Tumors

In adults, renal neoplasms account for 2% of all cases of malignant tumors. Renal cell carcinoma is the most common form, accounting for 80% to 85% of cases. Other less common renal cancers include transitional cell carcinoma, nephroblastoma, and sarcomas.

Renal cell cancer usually affects men older than age 50. Smoking, long-term use of phenacetin, and a family history of renal cell carcinoma may predispose a person to developing the disease.

Renal tumors are often initially surrounded by a fibrous covering called a pseudocapsule. If the tumor penetrates the pseudocapsule, the tumor could then extend into the perinephric fat and spread to adjacent structures, such as the liver, adrenal glands, pancreas, colon, and spleen. Metastasis may occur by way of the lymphatic system but usually occurs by way of venous drainage. Tumor thrombi may occur in the renal veins and the inferior vena cava. Some distant sites of metastases may be the lungs, the liver, bones, the brain, the adrenal gland, or the other kidney.

Transitional cell carcinoma affects the transitional epithelium that lines the hollow viscera of the urinary tract from the calices to the posterior urethra. The condition commonly appears between ages 50 and 80 and more often in men than in women. Risk factors include heavy smoking, phenacetin abuse, and prolonged exposure to aniline dyes or petroleum derivatives.

Squamous cell carcinoma may develop in the urinary tract from chronic irritation, urinary calculi, or schistosomiasis. Squamous cell carcinoma affects the bladder more often than the ureters or the collecting system, and often invades the urinary epithelium through the lamina propria and the muscularis. Once the muscularis is penetrated, the tumor can grow into adjacent tissues and spread rapidly through the lymph system.

⇨ Clinical signs

Signs and symptoms of renal cell carcinoma include hematuria, flank pain, flank mass, fever, weight loss, and varicoceles. Some patients may be seen initially for anemia, polycythemia, abnormal liver function, or polymyositis because the signs and symptoms of these syndromes are associated with renal cell carcinoma. Severe systemic coagulation disorders rarely occur secondary to renal cell carcinoma. (See "Case study: Renal cell carcinoma with embolization," page 270.)

Either macroscopic or microscopic hematuria is the most comon finding in transitional cell carcinoma. Pain may occur and is mainly the result of upper tract tumors that cause obstruction. A mass is infrequently palpated.

⇨ Radiographic findings

Renal cell carcinoma
With this tumor, excretory urography typically reveals:
• after I.V. contrast medium administration, a peripheral mass, a bulge, or an interruption in the renal contour and compression or displacement of the renal pelves or calyces
• changes in the axis of the kidney if the tumor is large
• impaired or absent kidney function.
Plain X-ray films typically show:
• a renal mass with calcium present.
Ultrasonography helps determine if the mass is a solid cyst,

Bladder and ureter transitional cell carcinoma

This film shows transitional cell carcinoma involving a 52-year-old woman's distal ureters. Contrast dye injected into the ureter using a percutaneously placed antegrade catheter ➔ reveals a strictured area ➤ involving the distal ureter and the ureterovesical junction ➔. The stricture was caused by the cancer.

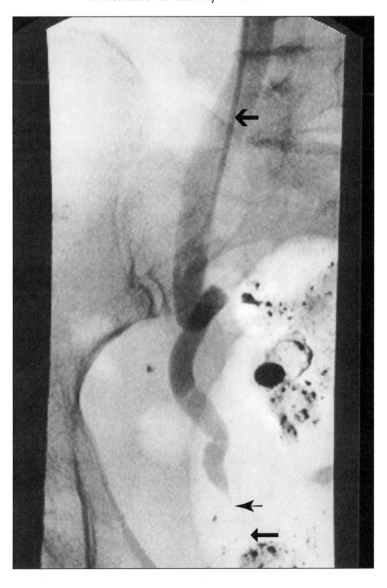

fluid-filled, or of indeterminate makeup.

CT scans may:
- differentiate a renal cyst from a tumor
- identify areas of necrosis within the mass (which appear as regions of low density)
- determine the shape and depth of the lesion wall (which is often irregular and thick)
- reveal stippled or irregular calcifications.

CT scanning also allows highly accurate staging of the tumor and helps guide the selection of treatment.

Angiography is used to determine vascularity and inferior vena cava involvement in carcinoma. Renal cell carcinomas typically show up as:
- hypervascular areas.

Transitional cell carcinomas of the ureters and collecting system

Excretory urography typically reveals:
- polypoid or flat tumors with an irregular outline rising from the wall of the collecting system, or a ureter producing obstruction and hydronephrosis (see *Bladder and ureter transitional cell carcinoma*)
- lucent filling defects.

Cystoscopy may identify bladder involvement, CT scanning identifies the tumor stage.

⇨ Treatment

Radical nephrectomy, the primary treatment for renal cell carcinoma, is the only curative treatment for stage I involvement. Palliative nephrectomy may be performed in patients who have marked hematuria, pain, hypercalcemia, and heart failure caused by arteriovenous shunting. Renal artery embolization may reduce tumor size and decrease blood loss during nephrectomy. Palliative radiation therapy may also be used. Chemotherapy has had mixed results but may be used for metastatic involvement. Tumor staging helps to determine the most effective treatment of transitional cell carcinoma. Cystoscopy and biopsy can aid in determining bladder-wall involvement. Surgical resection is the treatment of choice in such cases, with radiation and chemotherapy used palliatively, especially in metastatic disease.

Trauma

Trauma of the urinary tract may lead to disruption in urine formation and excretion, along with bleeding from the highly vascular kidneys. Prompt radiologic assessment is crucial in detecting life-threatening injuries and for preventing chronic impairment of urinary tract organs.

Renal injuries — blunt or penetrating — are classified as minor, major, or devastating. Approximately 80% to 85% of renal injuries are minor. These patients are hemodynamically stable, have negligible radiographic abnormalities, and are treated conservatively.

Major renal injuries account for 10% to 15% of renal trauma cases. Renal injuries are often associated with injuries to other organs. Patients may be treated conservatively but frequently experience severe sequelae without prompt surgical repair. Major renal injuries include urinoma, hematoma, arteriovenous fistula formation, and parenchymal fractures.

Devastating renal injuries require urgent surgical intervention to prevent irreparable damage. Such injuries include pedicle injury with vascular occlusion or tear, severance of the renal pelvis or ureter, and shattered kidney. Patients with those injuries are clinically unstable and frequently have multiple-system injuries. If the patient's condition permits, radiographic assessment of coexistent injuries is recommended prior to surgery.

Ureteral injury usually stems from penetrating or iatrogenic injuries. Injury from pelvic-cancer surgery or radiation therapy are most common. Severe traumatic injures may result in partial or complete severance of the ureters or in a tear at the ureterovesical junction.

Isolated bladder injuries are uncommon. Most patients experience accompanying pelvic fractures. Bladder injuries are classified as contusions or as intraperitoneal or extraperitoneal ruptures. Unrecognized ruptures may lead to reabsorption of urine from the peritoneal cavity.

⇔ Clinical signs

Patients may experience a variety of symptoms, depending on the site of injury and the degree of damage. Assessment of vital signs to detect blood loss and shock is imperative.

Hematuria may be present. A flank mass or bruise that gets larger may indicate hematoma.

Patients with acute bladder trauma may experience hematuria, pelvic pain, rigidity of the lower pelvic region, dysuria, and decreased urine output.

⇔ Radiographic findings

Most renal injuries can be evaluated by one of three procedures — excretory urography, CT scanning, or arteriography.
• Excretory urography identifies the degree of kidney function and areas of extravasation.
• Angiography reveals the degree of vascular injury present.
• CT scanning identifies the presence and degree of parenchymal injuries. It can also pinpoint bony fragments and shows their relationship to soft tissue, as well as detect minute extravasation of urine that contains contrast medium.
• Retrograde and antegrade ureterography identify problems with the ureters, such as partial or complete ureter severance or impairment of their lumens. Use of contrast medium may demonstrate the level of injury by identifying the presence or absence of extravasation outside the ureter. (See *View of a ureteral injury*, page 267.)
• Static cystography is the procedure of choice for evaluating traumatic bladder injuries. It identifies bladder ruptures, which appears as extravasation of contrast medium outside the bladder. It also shows bladder contusion as a crescent-shaped filling defect in the distended bladder wall or as a nondistensible segment of bladder wall.

⟿ Treatment

In most cases, renal trauma is best treated conservatively. Supportive therapy includes I.V. infusions, anti-inflammatory agents, steroids, prophylactic antibiotics, and alleviation of urinary obstruction. Surgical repair is reserved for severe cases of renal damage in which nephrectomy may prove necessary. Ureteral tears may be treated with retrograde stent placement or radiologically with percutaneous nephrostomy or antegrade stenting. (See *Ureteral stenting*, page 268.) Surgical ureteroplasty may be needed for complete transection. Cystoscopy will allow direct visualization of bladder trauma. Continuous bladder irrigation using urinary catheterization may ease bleeding and inhibit clot formation. Surgical resection and repair may be needed in severe cases.

Catheters, drains, and stents

A variety of catheters, percutaneous drains, or stents are used to manage GU tract problems.

Percutaneous nephrostomy, nephroureteral, and internal ureteral stents are indicated to relieve urinary obstruction, to divert urine flow to control fistulae, and to provide access for further manipulations, such as ESWL and dilatation of strictures. They may also be performed to gain specific measurements of urine output and anatomic morphology.

To prepare the patient for the procedure, the nurse should ensure that:
• informed consent has been obtained
• the patient has taken nothing-by-mouth
• all coagulation studies have been checked
• I.V. fluids are being administered
• prophylactic antibiotics are being administered.

I.V. analgesia and local anesthesia are used to decrease discomfort during the procedure, which is done with the patient lying prone. I.V. contrast dye may be administered to visualize the kidney and to provide a target during fluoroscopy. Ultrasonography may also be used to guide the needle into the col-

View of a ureteral injury

This X-ray film of the ureter of a 48-year-old man shows an iatrogenic ureteral injury. Contrast was introduced using percutaneous nephrostomy and revealed a transected ureter with extravasation of contrast ⇒ into the retroperitoneum. Note the guidewire ➤ placed just above the ureteral tear.

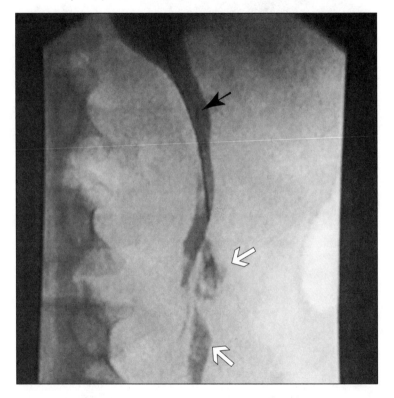

lecting system. One of the posterior calices is usually the preferred site for catheter placement.

A 22G needle is used to puncture the kidney and to inject the contrast dye. A series of guide wire-and-catheter manipulations are performed until a pigtail-loop catheter can be positioned in the renal pelvis. If access to the bladder is needed, the guide wire is manipulated into the ureter and then into the

Ureteral stenting

The guidewire and stent ➜ have been negotiated across the ureteral injury and into the bladder ⤍. The stent was removed after the ureter healed.

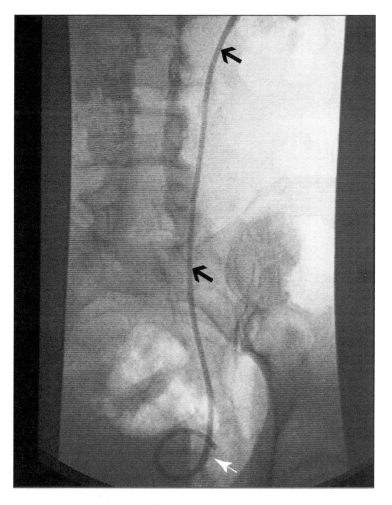

bladder. If external access is needed, a nephroureteral stent is placed. For internal placement, a ureteral stent is placed using pigtail loops positioned in the renal pelvis and bladder.

Nephrostomy catheters are made of a plastic radiopaque

Nephrostomy tube and stents

This film is of a 52 year-old woman with transitional cell carcinoma. It shows a left nephrostomy tube ⇒ placed temporarily and bilateral double pigtail internal stents ➤. Contrast medium is seen in the right collecting system and coursing down the right stent ⇒.

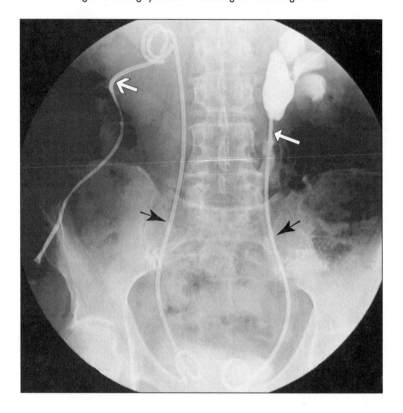

material. The pigtail-loop end of the catheter aids in stabilization within the renal pelvis. A series of holes in the loop facilitate urine drainage.

Ureteral stents are also made of a plastic radiopaque material and have double-J or loop configurations at each end. Holes are located in the renal loop and in the distal length and loop of the stent for urine drainage. (See *Nephrostomy tube and stents.*)

Case study: Renal cell carcinoma with embolization

Mr. Stone, a 42-year-old Air Force officer, was on duty in Alaska when he noticed some blood in his urine. Otherwise in good health, he noticed that he was losing weight although he wasn't on a diet. An initial IVP revealed a mass on his right kidney that was compressing the collecting system and distorting the renal outline. Tests also confirmed diminished function of the involved kidney.

After Mr. Stone was admitted to a local hospital, his condition rapidly declined and he was airlifted to another facility. He had massive hematuria and experienced hypotension and tachycardia. Blood studies revealed a hematocrit level of 24%, platelet count of 7,000/mm^3, and a prothrombin time (PT) of 27 seconds, findings that indicated disseminated intravascular coagulation. Mr. Stone received transfusions in an attempt to stabilize his condition.

Despite aggressive transfusions, however, his condition continued to deteriorate. An emergency CT scan revealed a large, necrotic, solid mass in the right kidney with no evidence of metastasis. Because Mr. Stone's condition was so unstable, doctors decided that surgery carried too high a risk and instead used angiography and embolization to treat the problem. Selective angiography revealed a large, encapsulated, highly vascular tumor typical of renal cell carcinoma.

After consulting with a urologist, Mr. Stone's radiologists elected to embolize the tumor with alcohol to achieve immediate and complete tumor ablation. Alcohol was infused into the renal artery using an occlusion balloon until there was no residual blood flow. Coils were then placed to mark the renal artery stump. (See *Placement of emboli coils.*)

Immediately after the procedure, Mr. Stone's hematuria resolved and his vital signs stabilized. By the next day, he was walking and his coagulation studies were returning to normal. His hematocrit level was stable at 32%; platelet count, at 97,000; and PT, at 17 seconds.

Two days later, Mr. Stone was taken to surgery for a right

Placement of emboli coils

This image is an angiogram of selective contrast medium injection into the right renal artery after alcohol infusion and placement of emboli coils ➔. Only a small adrenal branch ➤ remains patent. The remainder of the blood supply has thrombosed.

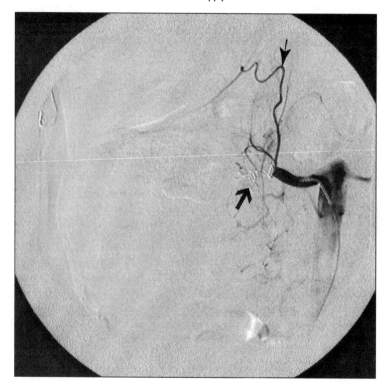

nephrectomy. Surgeons found no evidence of metastasis and were able to remove the tumor. Mr Stone was discharged 6 days later and within 6 weeks, was back at his duties with a prognosis for a full recovery.

Guide to patient care

This chart lists patient preparation and pretest and posttest care for various diagnostic-imaging tests of the GU system.

Test	Pretest care
Renal ultrasonography	• No food or fluid restrictions are required.
Renal computed tomography	• Restrict food for 4 hours before the test if the use of contrast medium is anticipated. Otherwise, foods and fluids are not restricted. • Administer a sedative if prescribed. • Note hypersensitivity to contrast medium on the patient's chart. • Have the patient remove metal objects that might obscure anatomic details.
Radionuclide renal imaging	• No food or fluid restrictions are required. • Withhold antihypertensive medications if ordered.

Posttest care	Patient instruction
• Make sure to remove all lubricating jelly from the patient's skin.	• Explain that this test is used to detect kidney abnormalities. • Inform the patient that he may be instructed to breathe deeply during the test. Explain that he may feel mild pressure as the transducer is passed over his skin.
• Resume the patient's usual diet.	• Explain to the patient that this test permits examination of the kidneys. • Inform the patient that he'll be positioned on an X-ray table so the scanner can take films of the kidneys. • Warn the patient that the scanner may make loud clacking sounds. • Inform the patient that he may experience transient adverse reactions such as a flushed feeling, a metallic taste, or a headache following contrast medium injection.
• As a radiation precaution, instruct the patient to flush the toilet immediately after voiding for the first 24 hours after the test.	• Explain that this test evaluates kidney structure, blood flow, and function and that several series of films of his bladder will be taken. • Inform the patient that the injection of radionuclide may cause a transient flushed feeling and nausea. • Emphasize that only a small amount of radionuclide is given and is usually excreted within 24 hours. • A pregnant female or a young child may receive supersaturated solution of potassium iodide (SSKI) 1 to 3 hours before the test to block thyroid uptake of iodide.

Test	Pretest care
Excretory urography	• Ensure that the patient is well hydrated until 8 hours prior to the test. Then restrict food and fluids. • Note hypersensitivity to contrast medium on the patient's chart. • Administer a laxative the night before the test, if necessary, to minimize poor resolution on X-ray films. • Have the patient put on a hospital gown and remove metal objects that might obscure anatomic detail in the scan. • Have the patient void before the test.
Kidney-ureter-bladder (KUB) radiography	• No food or fluid restrictions are required. • Have the patient remove jewelry and other metal objects and put on a hospital gown without metal snaps.
Voiding cystourethrography	• No food or fluid restrictions are required. • Note hypersensitivity to contrast medium on the patient's chart. • Administer a sedative just before the procedure if prescribed.

Posttest care	Patient instruction
• If a hematoma forms at the injection site, apply warm soaks. • Observe for delayed reactions to the contrast medium.	• Explain that this test helps to evaluate the structure and function of the urinary tract. • Inform the patient that he may experience a transient burning sensation and a metallic taste when the contrast medium is injected. Tell the patient to report other sensations he may experience. • Warn the patient that the X-ray machine may make loud clacking sounds.
• No posttest care is required.	• Explain that this test helps to detect urinary system abnormalities. • Determine childbearing status of female patients to reduce the risks of X-ray exposure to a pregnant female.
• Observe and record the time, color, and volume of the patient's voidings. Report hematuria if it persists after the third voiding. • Encourage the patient to drink large quantities of fluids, to reduce burning on urination and to flush residual contrast medium. • Monitor for chills and fever, which may be related to extravasation of contrast medium or to urinary sepsis.	• Explain that this test permits assessment of the bladder and the urethra. Tell him that a catheter will be placed into his bladder and that a contrast medium will be instilled into the bladder through the catheter. • Explain that X-rays of his bladder and urethra will be taken and that he may be asked to assume various positions. • Inform the patient that he may experience a feeling of fullness and an urge to void when the contrast dye is being instilled.

Test	Pretest care
Antegrade pyelography	• Restrict food and fluids for 6 to 8 hours before the test. • Administer antimicrobial drugs before and after the procedure if prescribed. • Note hypersensitivity to contrast medium on the patient's chart. • Administer a sedative just before the procedure, if prescribed.
Retrograde cystography	• No food or fluid restrictions are required. • Mark any hypersensitivity to contrast medium on the patient's chart.

Posttest care	Patient instruction
• Monitor vital signs every 15 minutes for the first hour, every 30 minutes for the second hour, and every 2 hours for the next 24 hours. • Check dressings with each vital sign check. Look for bleeding, hematoma, or urine leakage at the puncture site. For bleeding apply pressure. For hematoma, apply warm soaks. Report urine leakage or failure to void within 8 hours. • Monitor fluid intake and urine output for 24 hours. Report hematuria if it persists after the third voiding. • Watch for signs and symptoms of sepsis or extravasation of contrast medium—chills, fever, hypotension, rapid pulse, and rapid respirations. • Observe for and report signs that adjacent organs have been punctured—pain in the abdomen or flank and signs of pneumothorax (sudden onset of pleuritic chest pain, dyspnea, rapid pulse or rapid breathing, or decreased breath sounds on the affected side). • If a nephrostomy tube is inserted, check for patency and proper drainage. • Administer antibiotics and analgesics as ordered.	• Explain that this test allows radiographic examination of the kidneys. • Explain to the patient that after he receives a sedative and local anesthetic, a needle will be inserted into his kidney. • Explain that urine may be collected from the kidney for testing and that if necessary, a tube will be left in the kidney for drainage. • Inform the patient that he may feel mild discomfort during injection of a local anesthetic or a contrast medium and may feel transient burning and a flushed feeling from the contrast medium. • Warn the patient that the X-ray machine may make loud clacking sounds.
• Monitor vital signs every 15 minutes for the first hour, every 30 minutes for the second hour and then every 2 hours for up to 24 hours. • Record the time, color and volume of urine with each of the patient's voidings. Report hematuria that persists after the third voiding. • Watch for signs and symptoms of urinary sepsis due to urinary tract infection (chills, fever, elevated temperature, increased respiratory rate, or hypotension). Also watch for similar signs related to extravasation of contrast medium into the general circulation.	• Explain that this test permits an examination of the bladder. • Inform the patient that he may experience some discomfort when the catheter is inserted and when the contrast medium is instilled through the catheter. • Tell the patient he may hear loud clacking sounds as the X-ray films are being taken.

Test	Pretest care
Retrograde ureteropyelography	• Restrict food and fluids for 8 hours before the test if the use of general anesthesia is anticipated. • Administer medications before the test, as ordered.
Renal angiography	• Restrict food and fluids for 8 hours before the test. • Note hypersensitivity to contrast medium on the patient's chart. • Administer medications (usually a sedative and a narcotic) before the test, as ordered. • Have the patient put on a hospital gown and remove all jewelry and metal objects that might obscure anatomic detail on films. • Have the patient void before the test.

Posttest care

• Monitor vital signs every 15 minutes for the first 4 hours, then every hour for the next 4 hours, and then every 4 hours for 24 hours.
• Monitor fluid intake and urine output for 24 hours. Report gross hematuria or hematuria that persists after the third voiding. Also report lack of voiding within the first 8 hours after the test.
• Monitor urinary output if a urinary catheter is in place. An inadequate output may indicate that the catheter is obstructed and needs to be irrigated.
• Administer analgesics as ordered. Tub baths and increased fluid intake may reduce dysuria, which often occurs after this test.
• Watch for and report severe pain in the area of the kidneys, as well as signs of sepsis, such as chills, fever, and hypotension.

• Keep the patient flat in bed for at least 6 hours after the test.
• Check the patient's vital signs every 15 minutes for 1 hour, every 30 minutes for 2 hours, and then every 1 hour until stable.
• Monitor popliteal and dorsalis pedis pulses at least once an hour for 4 hours.
• Watch for bleeding and hematoma formation at the injection site. Check for bleeding each time you check vital signs.
• If bleeding occurs, apply pressure.

Patient instruction

• Explain that this test permits visualization of the urinary collecting system.
• Inform a female patient that she will be positioned on an examining table with her legs in stirrups.
• If awake, tell the patient he may feel pressure as the instrument is passed through the urethra. He may also feel pressure in the kidney area when the contrast medium is introduced.

• Explain that this test permits visualization of the kidneys, blood vessels, and functional units of the kidneys, and aids in the diagnosis of kidney disease and tumors.
• Inform the patient that he may experience transient discomfort (a flushed feeling, a burning sensation, nausea) during injection of the contrast medium.

Selected references

Davidson, A.J., and Hartman, D.S., eds. *Radiology of the Kidney and Urinary Tract,* 2nd ed. Philadelphia: W.B. Saunders Co., 1993.

Diseases. Springhouse, Pa.: Springhouse Corp., 1993.

Lewis, S.M., and Collier, I.C. *Medical Surgical Nursing, Assessment and Management of Clinical Problems,* 4th ed. St. Louis: Mosby–Year Book, Inc., 1992.

Marieb, E.N. *Human Anatomy and Physiology,* 3rd ed. Redwood City, Calif.: Benjamin/Cummings Publishing Co., 1995.

McCance, K.L., and Huether, S.E. *Pathophysiology: The Biological Basis for Disease in Adults and Children,* 2nd ed. St. Louis: Mosby–Year Book, Inc., 1994.

Taveras, J.M., and Ferrucci, J.T. *Radiology: Diagnosis-Imaging-Intervention,* vol. 2. Philadelphia: J.B. Lippincott Co., 1994.

7 Nervous system

The nervous system, the body's communications network, coordinates and organizes the functions of all other body systems. This intricate network has three divisions:
- the central nervous system (CNS), the control center, made up of the brain and spinal cord
- the peripheral nervous system, which includes nerves that connect the CNS to remote body parts and which relays and receives messages from these parts
- the autonomic nervous system, which regulates involuntary functions of organs.

Anatomy

The nervous system is one of the most complex phenomena known to humankind. This network of interlocking receptors and transmitters, along with the brain and spinal cord, forms a dynamic control system that controls and regulates every mental and physical function. From birth to death, the nervous system organizes the body's affairs: controlling the smallest action or reflex, expressing communication and instinct; and allowing introspection, wonder, abstract thought, and emotion. Major parts of the nervous system include neurons, the brain, and the spinal cord.

Neuron

Neurons are the basic building blocks of the nervous system. These highly specialized conductor cells receive and transmit electrochemical nerve impulses.

The neuron has a special, distinguishing structure. Delicate, threadlike nerve fibers extend from the central cell body and transmit signals; axons carry impulses away from the cell body and dendrites carry impulses to it. Most neurons have many

Structure of the neuron

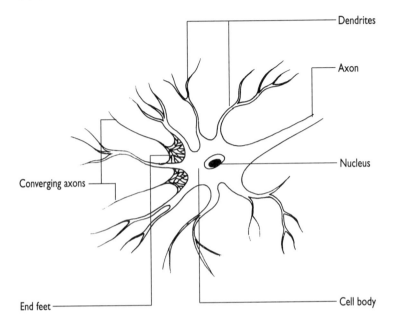

Dendrites

Axon

Nucleus

Converging axons

End feet

Cell body

dendrites but only one axon. (See *Structure of the neuron*.)

Sensory (afferent) neurons transmit impulses from special receptors to the spinal cord or brain. Motor (efferent) neurons transmit impulses from the CNS to regulate activity of muscles or glands. And interneurons (connecting or association neurons) shuttle signals through complex pathways between sensory and motor neurons. Interneurons account for 99% of all neurons in the nervous system and include most of the neurons in the brain.

Brain

The brain is the heart of the nervous system. It's a large, soft mass of nerve tissue housed in the skull. The brain's average weight is only 1.4 kg, but it consists of more than 12 billion neurons and 50 billion cells that help support neurons, called glial cells. The brain is protected and supported by the skull and the meninges, three closely associated connective membranes: the dura mater, the arachnoid, and the pia mater. The dura mater is the tough, white, fibrous outer sheath. The arachnoid membrane is the lace-like middle layer. The pia mater is the inner meningeal layer and consists of fine blood vessels held together by connective tissue. The pia mater is thin and transparent and clings to the brain and spinal cord, carrying branches of the cerebral arteries deep into the brain's fissures and sulci. Four ventricles, or spaces, are found inside the brain. These venticles produce cerebrospinal fluid, which helps protect the brain. Between the dura mater and the arachnoid membrane is the subdural space; the subarachnoid space lies between the pia mater and the arachnoid membrane.

Cerebrospinal fluid

Within the subarachnoid space and the brain's four ventricles is cerebrospinal fluid (CSF), a liquid composed of water and traces of organic materials, including protein, glucose, and minerals, plus lymphocytes to help prevent infection. The brain floats in CSF, which prevents the brain from crushing itself under its own weight. CSF also cushions the brain against external forces that might injure it. The fluid is also found in the spinal cord, which it also helps protect and nourish. CSF is formed from blood in capillary networks called choroid plexi, which are located primarily in the brain's lateral ventricles. CSF is eventually reabsorbed through hairlike vessels in dural sinuses on the surface of the brain.

Cerebrum

The cerebrum, the largest portion of the brain, houses the nerve center that controls sensory and motor activities and intelligence. The outer layer of the cerebrum, the cerebral cortex, consists of neuron cell bodies, or gray matter; the inner layers consist of axons, or white matter, plus basal ganglia, which control motor coordination and steadiness. The cerebral surface is deeply furrowed with elevations called gyri and depressions called sulci.

The longitudinal fissure divides the cerebrum into two hemispheres connected by a wide band of nerve fibers called the corpus callosum, which allows the hemispheres to communicate and to share learning and intellect. Both hemispheres don't share equally, though: One always dominates, giving that side control over the other. Because motor impulses descending from the brain cross in the medulla, the right hemisphere controls the left side of the body and the left hemisphere, the right side of the body. Several fissures divide the cerebrum into lobes, each of which is associated with specific functions.

Thalamus
The thalamus, a relay center below the corpus callosum, further organizes cerebral function by transmitting impulses to and from appropriate areas of the cerebrum. Besides its primary relay function, the thalamus is responsible for primitive emotional responses such as fear, and for distinguishing pleasant stimuli from unpleasant ones.

Hypothalamus
The hypothalamus, which lies beneath the thalamus, is the autonomic center that has connections with the brain, the spinal cord, the autonomic nervous system, and the pituitary gland. It regulates temperature, appetite, blood pressure, breathing, sleep patterns, and peripheral nerve discharges that occur with behavioral and emotional expression. It also partially controls pituitary gland secretions and stress reactions.

Cerebellum
Beneath the cerebrum, at the base of the brain, is the cerebellum. It's responsible for coordinating muscle movements with sensory impulses and maintaining muscle tone and equilibrium.

Brain stem
The brain stem houses cell bodies for most of the cranial nerves and includes the midbrain, the pons, and the medulla oblongata. With the thalamus and the hypothalamus, the brain stem makes up a nerve network called the reticular formation, which acts as an arousal mechanism. It also relays nerve impulses between the spinal cord and other parts of the

brain. The midbrain is the reflex center for the third and fourth cranial nerves and mediates pupillary reflexes and eye movements. The pons helps regulate respiration. The reflex center for the 5th through 8th cranial nerves, it assists in controling chewing, taste, saliva secretion, hearing, and equilibrium. The medulla oblongata influences cardiac, respiratory, and vasomotor functions.

Vasculature
Four major arteries—two vertebral and two carotid—supply the brain with oxygenated blood. These arteries originate in or near the aortic arch. The two vertebral arteries (branches of the subclavians) converge to become the basilar artery, which supplies the posterior brain. The common carotid arteries, which deliver 85% to 90% of the brain's blood supply, branch into the two internal carotid arteries. The internal carotids then divide to supply blood to the anterior and middle sections of the brain. These arteries interconnect through the circle of Willis at the base of the brain. This anastomosis ensures continual circulations to the brain despite interruption of any of the brain's major vessels. Most blood draining from the head is collected by the jugular veins.

Spinal cord
Extending for an average of 43 cm downward from the brain, through the vertebrae, to the second lumbar vertebra, is the spinal cord, a two-way conductor path between the brain stem and the peripheral nervous system. The spinal cord is also the reflex center for activities that don't require brain control, such as a knee-jerk reaction to the strike of a reflex hammer.

The spinal cord contains a mass of gray matter divided into horns. These horns are made up mostly of neuron-cell bodies that relay sensations and are needed for voluntary or reflex motor activity. The white matter surrounding the outer part of these horns consists of myelinated nerve fibers grouped functionally in vertical columns called tracts. (See *Inside the spinal cord*, page 286.) The thecal sac, a sheath of fibrous tissue, surrounds the spinal cord and helps protect it.

Inside the spinal cord

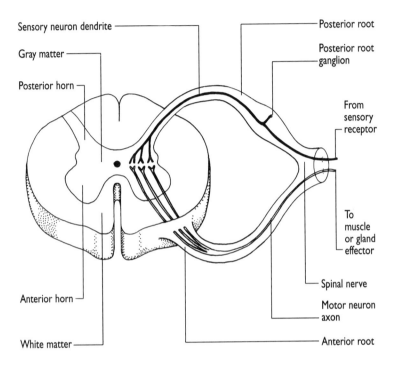

Sensory neuron dendrite

Gray matter

Posterior horn

Posterior root

Posterior root ganglion

From sensory receptor

To muscle or gland effector

Spinal nerve

Motor neuron axon

Anterior horn

White matter

Anterior root

The sensory, or ascending, tracts carry sensory impulses up the spinal cord to the brain, while motor, or descending, tracts carry motor impulses down the spinal cord. The brain's motor impulses reach a descending tract and continue through the peripheral nervous system by way of upper motor neurons.

Spine

The spine consists of 26 irregularly shaped bones called vertebrae, which surround and protect the spinal cord. It stretches from the brain stem, where it supports the skull, to the lumbar region of the back, where it anchors to the posterior surface of the pelvis and acts as a joint through which the weight of the torso is transferred to the legs. At the end of the spine is the tiny coccyx.

The spine has three major divisions: the 7 cervical vertebrae of the neck (C1-C7), the 12 thoracic vertebrae of the torso (T1-T12), and the 5 lumbar vertebrae of the lower back (L1-L5).

Imaging techniques

The soft and fibrous tissues of the nervous system may be examined with a variety of imaging techniques, depending on what is being examined and for what reason. (For information on patient preparation and care, see *Guide to patient care*, page 320 to 327.)

X-ray

Plain X-rays identify skull malformations, fractures, erosion, and thickening that may indicate tumors or increased intracranial pressure.

Computed tomography

Computed tomography (CT) scanning is usually the first technique used to view parts of the nervous system affected by acute or traumatic conditions. That's because the technique can display bony tissue as efficiently as it displays soft tissue and vascular structures. It also displays these structures clearly enough to differentiate them from one another when they appear in the same image. For that reason, a CT scan is the exam of choice to view acute intracranial hemorrhage. It's also used to identify intracranial tumors, arteriovenous malformation, and cerebral atrophy, calcification, edema, and infarction. I.V. injections of contrast media may enhance structures or particular pathologic disorders and aid in determining progression of healing. The procedure is invasive when contrast medium is used.

Magnetic resonance imaging

Because it produces images of the CNS in greater detail than a CT scan does, magnetic resonance imaging (MRI) is far better than CT scanning for detecting lesions of the brain stem and spinal cord. The test of choice for early detection of cerebral infarction and brain tumors, MRI can demonstrate demyelination disorders, such as multiple sclerosis, intraluminal clots and blood flow in arteriovenous malformations, and aneurysms.

Also, MRI has none of the hazardous side effects or possible complications associated with invasive techniques. It's contraindicated in patients with large metal clips, such as those used on aneurysms, because the magnet used to produce the image may dislodge the clip. It can also be a problem for patients who are claustrophobic, because the patient is confined within a tunnel-like chamber.

Transcranial Doppler ultrasonography

This noninvasive technique assesses intracerebral blood flow. Its use in detecting vascular spasm has led to a quicker intervention in this potentially fatal complication of aneurysm surgery than was possible before the technique was developed. Another form of transcranial Doppler ultrasonography, called color flow Doppler ultrasonography, is useful in screening patients for carotid artery stenosis.

Nuclear medicine

Nuclear brain scans are a relatively safe way of assessing blood flow in the brain and are used to determine brain function of patients in whom brain death is suspected. Studies of intercerebral shunts, known as shuntograms, have been done with the injection of an isotope into the cerebral shunt.

Single-photon emission computed tomography (SPECT), a type of nuclear medicine scan, uses an iodinated radiotracer to study blood flow and metabolism. SPECT scanning is useful in the study of stroke, epilepsy, and dementia.

Myelography

This technique is used to diagnose some spinal abnormalities, such as stenosis, nerve-root compression, herniations, and tumors in patients unable to have MRI or when MRI studies need confirmation. A myelogram is performed by inserting a needle into the thecal sack—the sheath around the spinal cord—and injecting a radiopaque contrast medium to show the spinal cord and canal. A cervical or lumbar puncture is the usual entry point.

Interventional radiology

In cerebral angiography, a catheter is inserted into an artery—usually the femoral artery—and indirectly threaded up to the carotid artery. Then, a radiopaque dye is injected to allow X-ray visualization of the cerebral vasculature.

Sometimes, the catheter is threaded directly into the brachial or carotid artery. This test can show cerebrovascular abnormalities and spasms, plus arterial changes from tumors, arteriosclerosis, hemorrhage, aneurysms, or blockage from a cerebrovascular accident (CVA).

Pathophysiology

Vascular disorders of the brain may have far-reaching, sometimes catastrophic, effects on the lives of the people afflicted with them. Cerebrovascular ischemia and infarction, or stroke, is the third leading cause of death in the United States. Intracranial aneurysms that rupture and bleed are another major source of neurologic injury. Also, trauma to the brain may lead to a hematoma that can deprive sensitive tissues of oxygen and other nutrients.

Cerebrovascular accident

Also known as stroke, CVA is a sudden impediment of flow in one or more of the brain's blood vessels. CVA interrupts or diminishes oxygen supply and commonly damages or kills brain tissue. The sooner circulation returns to normal after a CVA, the better chances are for a person's complete recovery. About half of people who suffer a CVA, however, are permanently disabled. The same number of CVA victims experience a recurrence of CVA.

Even though stroke is the third leading cause of death among adults in the United States, the death rate from the disorder has fallen more than 50% in the last four decades, mostly because of increased education about risk factors and better control of hypertension. Although CVA mostly affects older adults, it can strike people of any age and occurs most commonly in men.

CVAs are classified by their course of progression. The least severe is the transient ischemic attack (TIA), or little stroke, which results from a temporary interruption of blood flow, usually in the carotid and vertebrobasilar arteries. A reversible ischemic neurologic deficit (RIND) is a neurologic impairment that produces effects for more than 24 hours but less than 3 weeks. In a completed stroke, neurologic deficits are maximal at onset and last longer than 3 weeks. Major causes of CVA include cerebral thrombosis, embolism, and hemorrhage.

Thrombosis of a blood vessel is the most common cause of CVA in middle-aged and elderly people. Typically, the main site of the obstruction is the extracerebral vessels, but it's sometimes intracerebral.

Embolism, the second most common cause of CVA, can occur at any age. It usually develops rapidly—in 10 to 20 seconds—and without warning. In 75% of CVAs, the left middle cerebral artery is the site of the embolus. The embolus blocks blood flow in the affected artery and causes a densely ischemic area called the central focus, which is surrounded by a less dense ischemic area. Cells in the central focus are nearly always irreversibly damaged, unless they are quickly reperfused. The area surrounding the central focus usually remains viable for several hours. Quick-salvage therapies are aimed at saving these peripheral cells at risk of irreversible damage. Effects of CVA, such as edema, ischemia, and cell death, can be seen on imaging studies.

Hemorrhage, the third most common cause of CVA, may occur suddenly at any age. Such hemorrhage results from chronic hypertension or aneurysms that cause sudden rupture of a cerebral artery. Typically, active bleeding lasts less than an hour. Cerebral edema rapidly occurs and progresses for 1 to 2 days. The clinical course varies widely and 25% of victims die in the first 48 hours after the hemorrhage occurs.

➥ Clinical signs

Clinical features of CVA vary with the artery affected, the severity of the damage, and the extent of collateral circulation that develops to help compensate for decreased blood supply.

If the CVA occurs in the left hemisphere, it produces signs and symptoms on the right side of the body; if it occurs in the right hemisphere, signs and symptoms appear on the left side. A CVA that causes cranial nerve damage, however, produces signs of cranial nerve dysfunction on the same side as the hemorrhage.

Signs and symptoms include paresthesia, paresis, paralysis, visual disturbances, dysphagia, aphasia, coma, and death. The region affected and the length of time after the occurrence will dictate what symptoms will be seen. Symptoms may progress as edema forms in the damaged area. Most symptoms peak at 72 hours, if no new bleeding occurs.

➥ Radiographic findings

A CT scan is usually the first study performed when a CVA is suspected. A CT scan can diagnose or exclude intracerebral hemorrhage or identify an underlying structural lesion, such as tumor, arteriovenous malformation, or subdural hematoma that can mimic a stroke. It can also detect edema and such lesions as non-hemorrhagic infarctions and aneurysms.

CT scan findings in acute infarction evolve over time. Initial CT scans, for instance, may not detect nonhemorrhagic strokes less than 12 hours old. After 12 hours, increasing mass around the affected area, along with a wedge-shaped area of low density involving gray and white matter and corresponding to the injured territory, may be seen. (See *Subacute CVA in CT scans,* page 292.)

These other findings are consistent with CVA.

• Hemorrhagic strokes and intracerebral bleeds appear as radiodense areas within the brain matter. (See *CT scan of hypertensive hemorrhage,* page 294.)

• In the first few days, the blood-brain barrier remains

Subacute CVA in CT scans

These scans were taken of a 62-year-old man 4 days after onset of right hemiplegia. Figure A, performed without contrast medium, shows a wedge-shaped area of low density in the left hemisphere ◗. Also apparent is compression of the left ventricle → and a midline shift to the right. Figure B, performed using contrast medium, shows marked image enhancement of the area involved ◗.

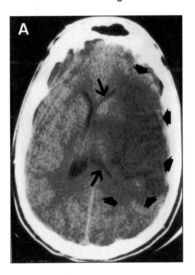

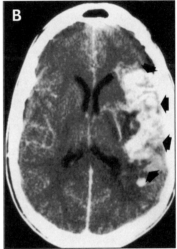

intact, so there is no image enhancement after I.V. contrast medium is injected. But 3 to 7 days after injury, blood-brain barrier permeability occurs and in most cases, the area around or inside the lesion appears enhanced after injection of I.V. contrast material.

• Patients who experience a TIA commonly have a normal CT scan.

• MRI allows evaluation of the lesion's location and size without exposing the patient to radiation.

• MRI findings may also be clearer than CT scan findings in a stroke's critical stage. For example, MRI images will show an absence of the normal blood flow as a lack of signal or blackness on the image of the thrombosed vessels and early edematous changes as increased signal (whiteness).

• MRI, however, doesn't distinguish among hemorrhage,

tumor, and infarction as well as CT scans do, but is superior in imaging the cerebellum and brain stem.

• Angiography details disruption or displacement of the cerebral circulation by occlusion or hemorrhage. It's the test of choice for examining the entire cerebral artery circulation. Angiography is not, however, traditionally performed to evaluate acute strokes. If plans are made to dissolve the clot with Urokinase, angiography is necessary to pinpoint and determine the extent of the clot and to plan therapy. Other studies, such as ultrasonography, are used to evaluate the carotid and vertebral arteries for a source of embolic strokes.

Other studies that may further define CVA include the following.

• Digital subtraction angiography evaluates the patency of cerebral vessels and identifies their position. It also detects and evaluates lesions and vascular abnormalities.

• Positron emission tomography provides data on cerebral metabolism and cerebral blood-flow changes.

• Single-photon emission tomography identifies cerebral blood flow and helps diagnose cerebral infarction.

• Transcranial Doppler studies examine the size of intracranial vessels and the direction of blood flow.

• Electroencephalography may detect reduced electrical activity in an area of cortical infarction. This test proves especially useful when CT scan results are inconclusive. It can also differentiate seizure activity from CVA.

⇔ Treatment

Aggressive, early management and treatment of CVA can improve prognosis. Prompt imaging with definitive diagnosis of the underlying cause directs therapeutic intervention. Medical management of CVA commonly includes physical rehabilitation, dietary and drug regimens to decrease risk factors, possible surgery, and care measures to help the patient adapt to specific deficits, such as speech impairment and paralysis.

Depending on the CVA's cause and extent, the patient may undergo a craniotomy to remove a hematoma, endarterectomy to remove atherosclerotic plaques from the inner arterial wall,

CT scan of hypertensive hemorrhage

This scan is from a 48-year-old man with acute onset of left-sided weakness and a blood pressure of 230/115 mm Hg. Taken without contrast medium, this scan reveals a high-density hematoma ➔ in the right basal ganglia. Blood has also spread to the right lateral ventricle ➔.

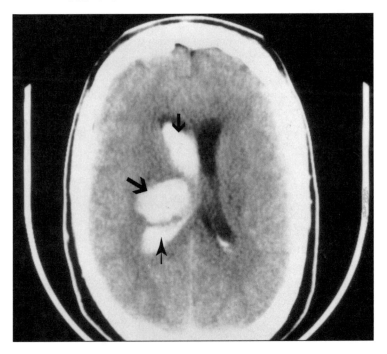

or extracranial-intracranial bypass to circumvent an artery that's blocked by occlusion or stenosis. Ventricular shunts may be necessary to drain CSF.

Medications useful in CVA include anticonvulsants, such as phenytoin or phenobarbital, to treat or prevent seizures; stool softeners, such as dioctyl sodium sulfosuccinate, to avoid straining, which increases intracranial pressure (ICP); corticosteroids, such as dexamethasone, to minimize associated cerebral edema; and analgesics, such as codeine, to relieve headache that may follow hemorrhagic CVA. Usually, aspirin is contraindicated in hemorrhagic CVA because it increases bleeding tendencies, but it may be useful in preventing TIAs.

Aneurysms

These localized dilations of a cerebral artery result from a weakness in the arterial wall. The most common form is the saccular (berry) aneurysm, a saclike outpouching in a cerebral artery. Most cerebral aneurysms occur at bifurcations of major arteries in the circle of Willis and its branches. (See *Common sites of cerebral aneurysm*, page 296.) An aneurysm can produce neurologic symptoms by exerting pressure on the surrounding structures such as the cranial nerves.

Cerebral aneurysms commonly rupture, causing subarachnoid hemorrhage (SAH). Sometimes, bleeding also spills into the brain tissue and forms a clot, which results in potentially fatal increases in ICP.

The prognosis is usually guarded, but depends on the patient's age and neurologic condition, other diseases present, and the extent and location of the aneurysm. About half of patients who suffer SAHs die immediately. With new and better treatment, however, prognosis is improving.

⮑ Clinical signs

Most intracranial aneurysms are asymptomatic until they rupture. When symptoms do appear, they include an unusually severe headache accompanied by nausea, vomiting and, commonly, loss of consciousness.

The patient or family member may report that the rupture of the aneurysm was preceded by a period of activity, such as exercise, labor and delivery, or sexual intercourse. The patient may also have a history of hypertension, infection, or head injury.

Occasionally, aneurysm rupture occurs as a slow leak, causing premonitory symptoms that last several days, such as headache, stiff back and legs, and intermittent nausea.

Other findings vary with the location of the aneurysm and the extent and severity of hemorrhage. Bleeding causes

Common sites of cerebral aneurysm

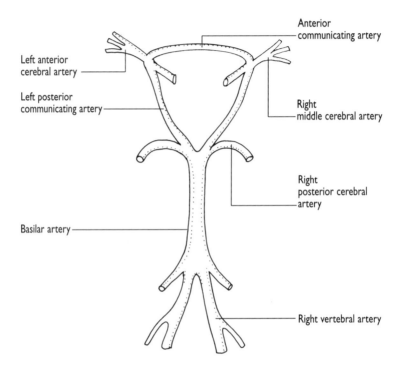

meningeal irritation, which can result in nuchal rigidity, back and leg pain, fever, restlessness, irritability, seizures, and blurred vision. If the aneurysm is adjacent to the oculomotor nerve, ptosis and vision disturbances may occur. If bleeding extends into the brain tissue, hemiparesis, unilateral sensory deficits, dysphagia, visual defects, and altered consciousness may occur. Lumbar puncture can detect blood in CSF, but is contraindicated if the patient shows signs of increased ICP.

⌖ Radiographic findings

A CT scan is the test of choice to diagnosis acute SAH. Here are the typical findings.
• Whiteness appears in the subarachnoid spaces.

• Most aneurysms arise in vessels of the circle of Willis or in the bifurcation of the middle cerebral artery. However, occasionally another vessel is involved.

• Blood usually fills the basal cisterns and sylvian fissures first. It may later mix with CSF and spread over the cerebrum, appearing as a feathery density throughout the sulci.

• SAHs older than a week may be hard to detect with a CT scan because blood may have cleared from the CSF. However, CSF analysis using lumbar puncture may help if imaging is inconclusive.

• A CT scan may reveal the SAH source, but angiography is usually required to find the source and guide therapy.

• Diagnosis of an aneurysm is usually made with a cerebral angiogram. In the test, each vessel is catheterized and studied to detect aneurysms.

• The goals of angiography include determining if an aneurysm is present, determining its location and size and whether there's more than one, evaluating the condition of the other cerebral circulation, and finding out whether there's a neck on the aneurysm, which may indicate rupture.

• Angiography finds a patent intracranial aneurysm that appears as a contrast-filled outpouching commonly rising from an arterial wall or bifurcation of a vessel.

• Skull X-rays may show calcification in the walls of a large aneurysm.

⇨ Treatment

Surgical clipping of unruptured aneurysms is the treatment of choice. The larger the aneurysm, the greater the potential for rupture. For ruptured aneurysms, the earliest surgical intervention is needed to prevent new incidents of bleeding.

When surgery poses too much risk (in very elderly patients or in those with serious heart, lung, or other major diseases), when the aneurysm is in a particularly dangerous location, or when vasospasm necessitates a delay in surgery, the patient may receive conservative treatment such as:

• bed rest in a quiet, darkened room, continued for 4 to 6

weeks if immediate surgery isn't possible
• avoidance of coffee and other stimulants
• avoidance of aspirin
• administration of codeine or other analgesic, as needed
• hydralazine or another antihypertensive agent if the patient is hypertensive
• a vasoconstrictor to maintain blood pressure at the optimal level (20 to 40 mm Hg above normal), if necessary
• phenobarbital or another sedative
• aminocaproic acid, a fibrinolytic inhibitor, to minimize the risk of new bleeding by delaying blood-clot lysis.

Antispasmodic drugs and intravascular volume expanders may improve outcomes. Interventional radiological techniques that may improve outcomes include intra-arterial infusions of vasodilators, such as papaverine, and intracranial balloon dilation. (See "Case study: Cerebral aneurysm with subarachnoid hemorrhage," page 315.)

Malignant tumors

Cancers of the nervous system are among the deadliest and most disfiguring. Involvement of speech and sense organs, along with effects on the CNS itself, can have an enormous impact on the patient's quality of life.

Malignant brain tumors cause CNS changes by invading and destroying tissue and by producing secondary effects— mainly compression of the brain, cranial nerves, and cerebral vessels as well as cerebral edema and increased ICP.

With an overall incidence of 5 per 100,000, malignant brain tumors account for about 2% of all deaths and 10% to 15% of all cancer deaths. In adults, the incidence of malignant tumors is highest between ages 40 and 60.

These tumors can occur at any age and are slightly more common in men than in women. In children, malignant brain tumors are among the most common causes of death. They typically occur up to age 12.

Types of malignant brain tumors include gliomas, meningiomas, and schwannomas.

Gliomas

Gliomas (which take their name from the inner brain cells where they originate) are the largest group of primary CNS tumors. Most gliomas are supratentorial—located above the covering of the cerebellum.

Types of gliomas include glioblastoma multiforme, astrocytoma, oligodendroglioma, and ependymoma. Often called *intra-axial* because they originate in the center of the brain, these tumor types account for up to 60% of brain tumors. (Metastatic lesions, which originate elsewhere in the body but spread to the CNS, account for the other 40%.)

Meningiomas

Meningiomas are the most common type of extra-axial tumors. (Extra-axial tumors are those that occur outside the brain tissue itself, arising in the subarachnoid, dural, epidural, or intraventricular spaces.) About 90% of meningiomas are supratentorial.

Schwannomas

These tumors are actually benign but are classified as malignant because of their growth patterns. They affect the craniospinal nerve sheath.

➡ Clinical signs

Clinical manifestations of malignant tumors vary widely, depending on tumor location and size. Signs may range from slightly decreased mental acuity to seizures. Stroke-like symptoms may be seen. Headache or other pain may occur initially, and then reappear as the tumor progresses.

Lumbar puncture findings may include increased CSF pressure, increased protein levels, decreased glucose levels, and occasionally, tumor cells in CSF.

➡ Radiographic findings

Plain X-rays, CT scans, MRI, and cerebral angiography help locate brain tumors.

Glioblastoma multiforme on MRI scan

This axial MRI image from a 51-year-old woman who presented with memory loss reveals a mass ▶ with marked white matter edema ➡.The tumor infiltrates across the midline and invades the corpus callosum ➤, which is typical of this disease.The lateral ventricles are compressed ➡.

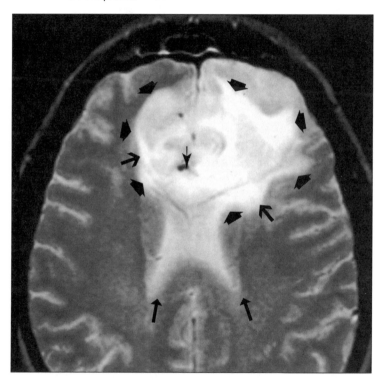

Glioblastoma multiforme

CT scans may reveal distortion of one lateral ventricle, with contralateral displacement of both lateral and third ventricles. (See *Glioblastoma multiforme on MRI scan*.)

Astrocytoma

This tumor's appearance varies with its degree of aggressiveness. Imaging techniques used to evaluate astrocytoma include

CT, MRI, and angiography. Here's what these techniques may show.

CT scans of aggressive astrocytoma reveal:
• a nonuniform, mass of mixed density
• compression and displacement of structure in scans without contrast medium (often)
• frequent good definition with use of intravenously injected contrast medium, with enhancement usually most prominent at the tumor margins (so-called rim enhancement in which the edges of the tumor are well defined)
• occasional diffuse infiltration and no discernible border
• varying degrees of cerebral edema, which causes low density in the brain tissue and compresses the ventricle and sulci
• frequently, a midline shift
• hemorrhage, if it has occurred in the tumor.

MRI images of aggressive astrocytomas may reveal:
• a poorly delineated lesion with intensity of the imaging signal ranging from white to dark gray in the tumor area
• a white core surrounded by a gray rim with peripheral dark fingerlike projections caused by edema that produces vascularity.

Angiograms usually show:
• astrocytomas as a mass, which causes normal vessels to be pushed away from their normal location
• tumor stain, in which contrast medium remains in the tomor region after the contrast medium has washed away
• a higher than normal number of blood vessels with irregularly tapered ends.

Meningioma

These tumors are usually denser than surrounding brain tissue. CT scan reveals:
• a sharply circumscribed round or smoothly lobulated mass adjacent to a dural surface
• calcification in 25% of tumors
• possible hyperostosis (overgrowth of adjacent bone)
• sometimes, invasion of the skull, with destruction of bone
• edema in adjacent brain tissue (60% of the time)
• marked enhancement ("lighting up") of the tumor when

MRI scans of meningioma

These MRI scans, done after administration of I.V. gadolinium, are of a 47-year-old woman who complained of a right-sided headache. Figure A, an axial scan, shows an extraaxial mass in the right cerebellar tentorium ◊. Note compression of the cerebellum ⇢ and brain stem ⟹. Figure B, a coronal scan, also shows a mass ◊ in the right cerebellum ⇢ and brain stem ⟹.

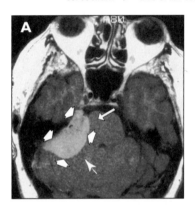
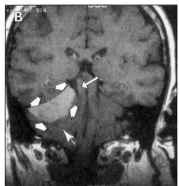

I.V. contrast medium is used.

MRI findings typically include:
• displacement of gray and white matter and a cleft or rim of CSF or vessels surrounding the mass and separating it from the brain tissue (see *MRI scans of meningioma*)
• edema, usually.

Angiogram findings include:
• a sunburst type of vascular enhancement seen clearly after intra-arterial injection of contrast dye
• the "mother-in-law" sign, a vascular blush that comes early and stays late, with contrast medium lingering in the tumor after it has been cleared from the rest of the vessels.

⟿ Treatment

Treatment goals are to locate the tumor, identify its type, remove it surgically, or decrease its mass with radiation or chemotherapy. For chemotherapy, many patients receive nitrosoureas. These antineoplastic agents cross the blood-brain barrier and allow other chemotherapeutic agents to cross. Intrathecal and intra-arterial administration maximize drug action.

Another treatment goal is to prevent neurologic impairment by preventing or managing increased ICP. This can be achieved with steroids, diuretics or, possibly, ventriculoatrial or ventriculoperitoneal CSF shunting.

Some patients receive anticonvulsants and narcotics to prevent and control seizures and manage pain. Treatments being explored for brain tumors include bone-marrow transplantation and hyperthermia.

Other treatments vary with the tumor's classification, radiosensitivity, and location.

Gliomas

Surgery is the treatment of choice for gliomas, followed by radiation and chemotherapy. Radiation combined with carmustine, lomustine, or procarbazine is more effective than radiation alone.

For some gliomas—especially medulloblastomas—surgery plus arterial embolization using percutaneous catheterization may be done. In the procedure, methotrexate or another antineoplastic drug is infused into the tumor site. Sometimes percutaneous catheterization is done to devascularize a tumor before surgery.

For low-grade cystic cerebellar astrocytomas, surgical resection often permits long-term survival. For other astrocytomas, treatment involves repeated surgery, radiation therapy, and CSF fluid shunting. Radiation works best in radiosensitive astrocytomas.

Treatment for two other types of gliomas, oligodendrogliomas and ependymomas, includes surgical resection and radiation therapy.

Meningiomas

These tumors require surgical resection. Operative mortality may reach 10% for large tumors.

Schwannomas

Microsurgery allows complete resection of schwannomas along with facial nerve preservation. Radiation follows.

Spinal tumors

Spinal tumors are rare compared to intracranial tumors. Tumors involving the spinal cord may be primary, such as astrocytoma or ependymoma. These tumors may also be secondary, or metastatic.

Spinal tumors are classified by location. They may be extramedullary (occurring outside the spinal cord) or intramedullary (occurring within the cord). Most extramedullary neoplasms are metastatic, usually arising from tumors of the breast, lung, or prostate.

Astrocytomas account for 40% of intramedullary spinal lesions and generally appear in patients ages 30 to 50. Usually, the neck and chest are involved. Astrocytomas are generally large and involve the entire diameter of the cord. Usually, they're infiltrative and nonresectable.

Ependymomas make up about 60% of intramedullary malignant spinal cord tumors and generally affect patients ages 40 to 50. Typically, the terminal spinal cord is involved. Ependymomas are well-circumscribed, noninfiltrating tumors with a tendency to hemorrhage. Most can be resected.

⇨ Clinical signs

Spinal cord tumors grow slowly and the spinal cord adjusts over time to the presence of the tumor. It may be several years between tumor genesis and onset of symptoms, and another 2½ years until diagnosis.

These tumors produce back pain, weakness, and muscle atrophy as the spinal cord is compressed, which leads to ischemia. Patient history may reveal pain most severe over the tumor or radiating around the trunk or down a limb on the affected side. Few measures relieve the pain, not even bed rest. Physical examination may find neurologic deficits, including contralateral loss of sensation to pain, temperature, and touch.

These losses are less obvious to the patient than functional motor changes.

Lumbar puncture reveals clear yellow CSF, caused by increased protein levels if the flow is completely blocked by a growth. If the flow is partially blocked, protein levels rise but the fluid appears only slightly yellow in proportion to the CSF protein level. A Papanicolaou test of the CSF may show malignant cells of metastatic carcinoma.

⇨ Radiographic findings

MRI is the test of choice to detect spinal cord lesions. Its capacity to produce images in sagittal, axial, and coronal planes, plus its high resolution of tissue differentiation, make it superior to CT scanning in detecting spinal cord lesions.

MRI of spinal cord neoplasms presents three general characteristics:
- a diffusely or focally enlarged spinal cord
- abnormal signal intensity
- bright enhancement with contrast material. (See *Spinal tumor*, page 306.)

CT scanning may show:
- bone erosion from extradural lesions
- intradural lesions.

Myelography identifies the level of a lesion by outlining the tumor if the tumor partially obstructs the progress of the contrast medium. However, this radiographic technique is dangerous when the spinal cord is almost completely compressed because withdrawn or escaping CSF will allow the tumor to exert greater pressure against the spinal cord.

Myelography may reveal:
- a mass in the spinal cord
- a mass displacing or compressing the spinal cord or thecal sac.

Plain X-rays will show:
- distortions of the intervertebral foramina
- changes in the vertebrae or collapsed areas in the vertebral body

Spinal tumor

This sagittal MRI is of a 50-year-old woman who developed increasing lower-extremity weakness and incontinence. It reveals an intradural extramedullary nodular mass → typical of meningioma. Note compression of the spinal cord →.

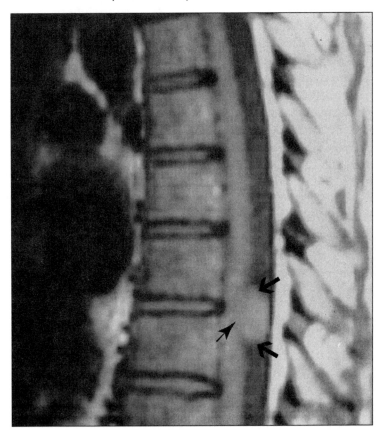

 • localized enlargement of the spinal canal, indicating an adjacent blockage.

Radioisotope bone scan demonstrates:

 • metastatic invasion of the vertebrae by detecting a characteristic increase in osteoblastic activity.

⮌ Treatment

Surgical resection is usually the first line of treatment for primary spinal cord lesions, if imaging results suggest that resectability is possible. Cure is often possible, especially for meningiomas and nerve sheath tumors. Laminectomy may be done for primary tumors that produce spinal-cord compression. If the tumor progresses slowly or is treated before the cord degenerates from compression, symptoms are likely to subside and function may return.

In a patient with metastatic carcinoma or lymphoma who suddenly experiences complete transverse myelitis with spinal shock, functional improvement is unlikely, even with treatment. Prognosis for this patient is poor.

Radiation therapy can usually shrink the tumor but is usually palliative. Relief of pain and restoration of function are the primary therapeutic goals after resection. Steroid therapy is used to shrink edema-related tumors that may cause further cord compression and ischemia.

If the patient has rapid-onset incomplete paraplegia, emergency surgical decompression may save cord function. Steroid therapy may control edema until surgery.

Partial removal of intramedullary gliomas, followed by radiation therapy, may temporarily ease symptoms. Metastatic extradural tumors can be controlled with radiation therapy, analgesics and, in hormone-mediated tumors (breast and prostate), appropriate hormone therapy.

Transcutaneous electrical nerve stimulation (TENS) may relieve radicular pain from spinal cord tumors and is a useful alternative to opioid analgesics.

Trauma

Fractures

Most head and spine fractures are caused by motor vehicle accidents. In older people, falls also account for many skull and vertebral fractures. Blunt trauma from violent acts is another significant source of skull and spine injury.

Skull fractures

Because the first concern with a skull fracture is possible damage to the brain rather than the fracture itself, the injury is considered a neurologic condition. Symptoms reflect the severity and extent of the head injury.

Skull fractures may be simple (closed) or compound (open) and may displace bone fragments. They're also described as linear, comminuted, or depressed. A linear, or hairline, fracture doesn't displace structures and seldom requires treatment. A comminuted fracture splinters or crushes the bone into fragments. A depressed fracture pushes the bone toward the brain; it's serious only if it compresses underlying structures.

Skull fractures also are classified according to location. A basilar fracture occurs in the anterior or middle fossa at the base of the skull and involves the cribriform plate and frontal sinuses.

Most skull fractures are caused by blunt trauma and usually are associated with other head wounds, such as abrasions, contusions, and lacerations. Motor vehicle accidents, falls, and beatings are the leading causes of skull fracture.

⮎ Clinical signs

Symptoms of skull fracture depend on the region and severity of the injury. Minor injuries may feature headache, scalp laceration, ecchymosis, edema, and bleeding. Severe injuries may cause stupor, unconsciousness, hemorrhage, and coma.

CSF leakage from the ear or nose may accompany basal skull fractures. There may also be bleeding in the nose, pharynx, or ears, under the conjunctivae or periorbital skin ("raccoon's eyes"), and behind the eardrum. Neurologic changes are an indication of cerebral injury or ischemia from edema.

⮎ Radiographic findings

CT scanning is the primary imaging technique in detecting skull injury. This powerful diagnostic tool can:
• assess bone fractures

• detect early signs of cerebral hemorrhage and evidence of mass effect and increased pressure on the brain

• show skull fractures as breaks in skull continuity that may show displacement of brain matter or associated signs of hemorrhage. (See *Skull fracture in CT scan*, page 310.)

Plain X-rays will detect skull fractures. Look for these signs:

• irregular radiolucent lines

• a C-shaped density produced by overlapping fragments (a depressed fracture).

Angiography locates:

• vascular disruptions from internal pressure or injury.

MRI and radioisotope scan disclose:

• intracranial hemorrhage from ruptured blood vessels.

⤳ Treatment

Conservative therapy is the usual course for treating closed skull fractures. Bed rest and supportive I.V. fluids are prescribed and frequent neurologic status checks are performed to monitor changes in function. Steroids may be used to treat or prevent cerebral edema. Analgesics should be used judiciously; otherwise they could mask changes in the patient's neurologic status.

Surgical intervention may be needed to remove blood clots and relieve pressure on the brain or to repair damage from depressed or comminuted skull fragments.

Severe fault fractures, especially depressed fractures, usually require craniotomy for evaluation or removal of fragments that have been driven into the brain and for extraction of foreign bodies and necrotic tissue. This reduces the risk of infection and further brain damage. Cranioplasty follows the use of tantalum mesh or acrylic plates to replace the removed skull section. The patient commonly requires antibiotics. With profound hemorrhage, the patient may also need blood transfusions.

A basilar fracture necessitates immediate administration of prophylactic antibiotics to prevent meningitis from CSF leaks. The patient also needs close observation for secondary

Skull fracture in CT scan

This CT scan is of a 28-year-old man who lost consciousness after a fight. Performed without contrast medium, it shows a highly dense collection of blood in the epidural space ▶ due to a temporal bone fracture. The collection of blood causes compression of the brain and a midline shift. Note the displaced third → and lateral ➤ ventricles.

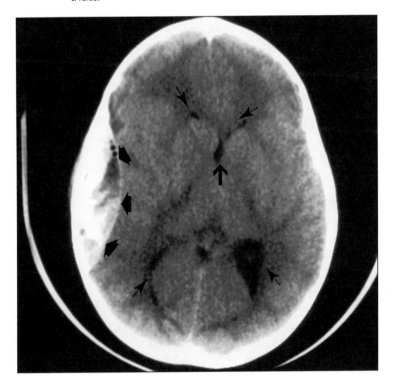

hematomas and hemorrhages. If they develop, surgery may be necessary.

A patient with a basilar or vault fracture also requires I.V. or I.M. dexamethasone to reduce cerebral edema and to minimize brain tissue damage. Careful monitoring of fluids and assessing for signs of cerebral edema are mandatory to prevent irreparable ischemic damage.

Spinal injuries

Spinal injuries occur with more-than-normal, or excessive, movement of the section of the spine involved, or by compactional or rotational force. These injuries can be classified into four categories:

• Flexion. Hyperflexion causes fracture or dislocation of vertebral bodies, such as disks or ligaments. This type of injury is common in the cervical and thoracic spine and at the thoracolumbar junction.

• Extension. Hyperextension of the spine causes fracture and dislocation of the posterior elements, such as the spinous processes, transverse processes, laminae, pedicles, or posterior ligaments. Hyperextension injuries are common in the cervical region.

• Compression. Vertical compression results in shattering, or burst, fractures. Cervical burst fractures are common diving injuries; thoracolumbar fractures are common jumping injuries.

• Rotation. Forces exerted on the spine during rotation result in rupture of supporting ligaments and in fractures. These injuries are most often seen with extension and flexion injuries.

Most spinal injuries occur at vertebrae C1, C2, C4, or C6, and at vertebrae T11 through L2 because these are the most mobile parts of the spine.

⮑ Clinical signs

Acute back pain and neurologic impairment are the usual signs of spinal fractures. Depending on the fracture level, symptoms range from paresthesia, paralysis, and pain to loss of voluntary sphincter control. The patient may also complain of muscle spasm and back or neck pain that worsens with movement.

In cervical fractures, tenderness may be present. In dorsal and lumbar fractures, pain may radiate to other body areas such as the legs.

Lumbar vertebral fractures

This anteroposterior projection X-ray of the lumbar spine of a 20-year-old man shows a transverse fracture through **L2** involving the body and both transverse processes ➔.

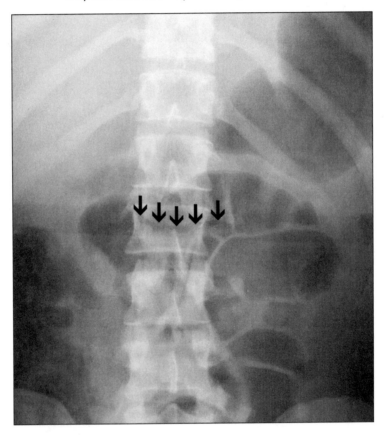

◔ Radiographic findings

• CT scanning best reveals spinal injuries and fractures. Bony fragments, for instance, may be identified in relationship to soft tissues.

• MRI is best for defining spinal cord lesions or injuries of the intervertebral disk or ligaments.

• Plain X-rays of the cervical and thoracolumbar region are usually the first studies done to rule out fractures after blunt trauma or motor vehicle accidents. (See *Lumbar vertebral fractures.*) Many of these patients arrive at the hospital in immobilization devices such as cervical collars until presence or absence of spinal fractures or injuries is determined.

⮌ Treatment

Conservative therapy is prescribed unless spinal cord injury is apparent. Spinal stabilization is usually the primary treatment goal until healing occurs. Surgery is reserved for injuries that may cause cord damage or to relieve cord compression. Antiinflammatories, analgesics, and steroids, along with other supportive measures, are used to promote healing.

Herniated disk

Also known as herniated nucleus pulposus, or a slipped disk, a herniated disk occurs when all or part of the nucleus pulposus — an intervertebral disk's gelatinous center — extrudes through the disk's weakened or torn outer ring (the annulus fibrosus). The resultant pressure on spinal nerve roots or on the spinal cord causes back pain and other symptoms of nerve-root irritation.

About 90% of herniations affect the lumbar and lumbosacral spine; 8% occur in the cervical spine; and 1% to 2% in the thoracic spine. The most common site for herniation is the space between vertebrae L4 and L5.

⮌ Clinical signs

Herniated lumbar disks cause back pain, with associated buttock and leg pain along the sciatic nerve. Results of the straight leg–raise test may be positive. Reflexes may be diminished or absent, and numbness and tingling may occur in the arms and legs. Motor weakness indicates severe involvement.

Herniated disk

These MRI scans are of a 33-year-old man with back pain that radiated down his left leg. The scan of the sagittal plane shown in figure A reveals loss of the normal bright signal in the L4-5 disk area ⚹. The L5-S1 disk material herniates into the spinal canal, displacing and compressing nerve roots ⇒. Figure B shows an axial image at L5-S1 with the disk material ⇒ compressing the bright, fluid-filled thecal sac on the left and obliterating the left nerve root. Note the normal right nerve root ⇾.

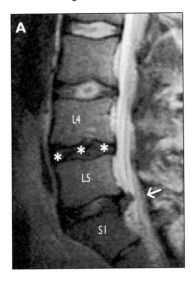

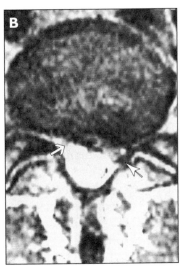

⇨ Radiographic findings

• CT scanning, CT myelography (a CT scan with intrathecal injection of contrast medium), and MRI can all accurately diagnose herniated disks.

• CT scans show a soft tissue mass with thecal-sac displacement.

• CT myelograms reveal an extradural mass caused by herniation and show the herniation's relationship to the spinal cord and nerve roots.

• MRI shows focal, asymmetric protrusions beyond the confines of the annulus. It reveals the herniation and its relationship to soft tissues. The annular tear may also be seen. (See *Herniated disk.*)

• X-ray studies of the spine are essential to show degenerative changes and to rule out other abnormalities. Films may not show a herniated disk because even marked disk prolapse may show up as normal on an X-ray.

• Myelography can pinpoint the level of the herniation and depict displacement of the contrast-filled thecal sac; elevation, deviation, or amputation of the root sleeve; and edema.

• Electromyography confirms nerve involvement by measuring electrical activity of muscles innervated by the herniated disk.

⮫ Treatment

A conservative approach may be tried first to manage a herniated lumbar disk. Other treatments include bed rest, pelvic traction, heat, physical therapy, anti-inflammatories, analgesics and muscle relaxants.

Surgery is used if conservative management fails and progressive neurologic impairment occurs. Spinal fusion may be necessary in the case of vertebral instability.

Case study: Cerebral aneurysm with subarachnoid hemorrhage

Mrs. Drake, age 47, was admitted to a hospital with what she described as the worst headache of her life. A CT scan revealed diffuse SAH. She was transferred to another hospital and admitted to the intensive care unit (ICU).

There, SAH protocols were instituted, consisting of bed rest, frequent vital-sign and neurologic-function checks, I.V. fluid administration, and administration of Decadron, Pepcid, Dilantin, Nimotop, and antihypertensive agents. Mrs. Drake was stabilized. Her neurologic function was intact, but she

Angiogram of an aneurysm

This lateral-view, left internal carotid angiogram reveals an aneurysm arising posteriorly from the left internal carotid artery at the origin of the posterior communicating artery ➜.

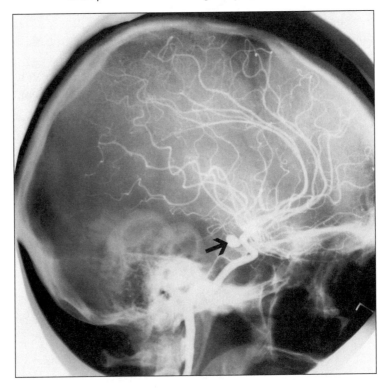

exhibited mild lethargy. Her speech was normal and her headache was treated with I.V. fentanyl.

A cerebral angiogram revealed a large aneurysm of the left posterior communicating artery. (See *Angiogram of an aneurysm*.) Surgery was scheduled.

Mrs. Drake's aneurysm was clipped without complications. She was returned to the ICU, where she was observed closely for signs of neurologic impairment. The next morning, Mrs. Drake was awake and alert. She continued recovering un-eventfully for the next 3 days. A routine follow-up angiogram

Postoperative angiogram

This lateral projection of the left internal carotid artery reveals no filling of the aneurysm. Note the aneurysm clip ➔ and scalp staples ➔.

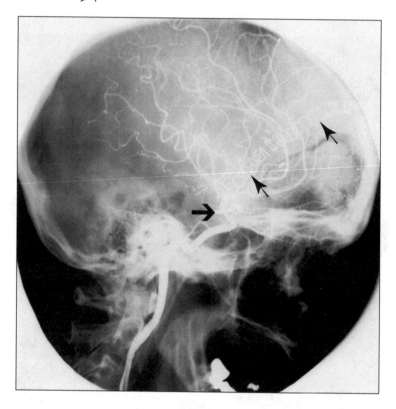

showed complete aneurysm clipping with minimal left internal carotid spasm. (See *Postoperative angiogram*.) She was doing well, aside from a slight short-term memory lapse, and was transferred to the surgical ward, with plans for discharge in 2 days.

But after 5 days, while being prepared for discharge, Mrs. Drake suddenly developed right-hand weakness. A CT scan showed only postoperative changes, without evidence of new bleeding or other problems.

Cerebral spasm

This anteroposterior view from a left internal carotid angiogram shows severe spasm in the anterior cerebral artery ➔ and the middle cerebral artery ➤. Serial films showed slow flow. Note the clip ⟶ and cranial defects ▶.

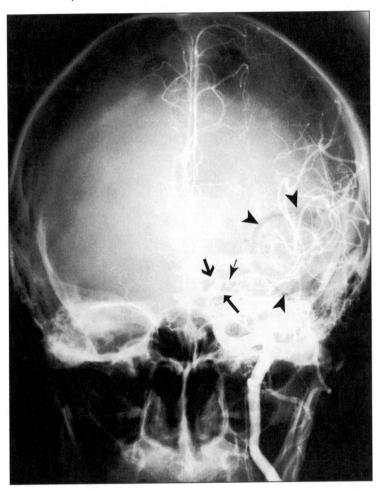

A transcranial Doppler ultrasonogram showed changes in intracranial-arterial velocities consistent with left middle cerebral artery spasm. A volume expander was ordered.

Mrs. Drake's condition continued to deteriorate, with slight aphasia, lethargy, mild right-side facial droop, and continued right-arm weakness. She was transferred back to the ICU for an aggressive antivasospasm regimen that included placement of a pulmonary artery catheter, administration of volume expanders, and a dopamine drip to maintain her blood pressure.

A cerebral angiogram revealed severe spasm of the left internal carotid artery's A1 and M1 branches. (See *Cerebral spasm.*) The left internal carotid artery was catheterized and the subselective middle cerebral and anterior communicating arteries were infused with 300 mg of papaverine over 1 hour.

Marked improvement of the vessels and Mrs. Drake's condition were noted. Balloon angioplasty of the left middle cerebral artery and internal carotid artery was accomplished.

Mrs. Drake left the angiography suite markedly improved, with nearly complete resolution of aphasia, lethargy, and right-arm weakness. The antivasospasm regimen was continued for the next 3 days, with tapering of medications. Transcranial Doppler studies were done daily to track blood flow.

Mrs. Drake left the ICU 4 days after angioplasty in stable condition. Although she had a slight residual neurologic deficit, she went home 14 days after the initial event with hope of a full recovery.

Guide to patient care

This chart lists patient preparation and pretest and posttest care for various diagnostic-imaging tests of the nervous system.

Test	Pretest care
Intracranial computed tomography	• No food or fluid restrictions are required unless the use of contrast medium is anticipated. In that case, have the patient fast for 4 hours before the test. • Administer a sedative, if prescribed. • Note hypersensitivity to contrast medium on the patient's chart. • Have patient put on a hospital gown and remove all metal objects that might obscure anatomic details in the scan.
Intracranial magnetic resonance imaging (MRI)	• No pretest food or fluid restrictions are required. • Administer sedation if patient suffers from claustrophobia. • Have the patient remove all metal objects, including jewelry, hairpins, and watches. Ask if he has any surgically implanted metal joints, pins, clips, valves, pumps, or pacemakers that could be attracted by the strong MRI magnet. If he does, he will not be able to undergo the test.

Posttest care	Patient instruction
• Observe for residual adverse reactions including headache, nausea, and vomiting. • Resume the patient's usual diet.	• Explain that this test permits assessment of the brain structures. • Tell the patient he will be placed on a moving X-ray table and that his head will be immobilized and his face uncovered. • Inform the patient that the X-ray machine makes loud clacking sounds. • If a contrast medium is used, tell the patient that he may feel flushed and warm and may experience a transient headache, a salty taste, or nausea and vomiting after the contrast medium is injected.
• Observe for postural hypotension if the procedure takes longer than normal.	• Explain that this test assesses the status of bones and soft tissue. • Explain that the test is not painful and involves no exposure to radiation from the scanner, but a radioactive contrast medium may be used, depending on the type of tissue being studied. • Ask the patient if he suffers from claustrophobia. If so, he may require sedation. • Tell the patient that he will hear the scanner clicking, whirring, and thumping. • Reassure the patient that he will be able to communicate.

Test	Pretest care
Transcranial Doppler studies	• No pretest food or fluid restrictions are required.
Spinal computed tomography	• Restrict food for 4 hours before the test if the use of contrast medium is anticipated. Otherwise, no food or fluid restrictions are required. • Administer a sedative if prescribed. • Note hypersensitivity to contrast medium on the patient's chart. • Have the patient remove metal objects that might obscure anatomic detail in the scan.

Posttest care	Patient instruction
• Make sure to remove all lubricating jelly from the patient's skin.	• Explain that this test measures the velocity of blood flow through cerebral blood vessels, detects the progression of cerebral vasospasm, and determines whether collateral blood flow exists. • Explain that the test is not painful but that he will feel pressure where the transducer is pressed against the skin. • Tell the patient that he may be asked to turn from side to side and to breath deeply.
• No posttest care is required if the procedure was performed without contrast enhancement. • Resume the patient's usual diet if contrast medium was used.	• Explain that this test permits visualization of the spine. • Tell the patient that he will be positioned on an X-ray table and that the scanner will make loud clacking sounds as it rotates. • Inform the patient that he may experience transient adverse effects, such as a flushed feeling, a metallic taste, and a headache following contrast medium injection.

Test	Pretest care
Myelography	• Restrict food and fluid for 8 hours before the test. • Note hypersensitivity to contrast medium on the patient's chart. • Notify the radiologist if patient has a history of epilepsy or of phenothiazine use. • Administer a cleansing enema before the test, if ordered. • Administer sedation and an anticholinergic as prescribed. • Have the patient remove jewelry, metal objects, and other objects that might obscure anatomic details in the film.
Skull radiography	• No pretest food or fluid restrictions are required. • Have the patient remove glasses, dentures, jewelry, and other metal objects that might obscure anatomic detail in the films.

Posttest care

- If the contrast dye metrizamide was used, tell the patient to remain in bed for 12 to 16 hours. Keep the head of the bed elevated for the first 6 to 8 hours.
- If an oil-based contrast medium was used, have the patient remain flat for 6 to 24 hours.
- Encourage the patient to drink extra fluids and void within 8 hours of the test.
- Resume the patient's usual diet and activity the day after the test.
- Monitor for radicular pain, fever, back pain, or signs of meningeal irritation, such as headache, irritability, or a stiff neck. If those signs occur, keep the room dark and quiet and administer an analgesic or antipyretic, as ordered.

- No posttest care is required.

Patient instruction

- Explain to the patient that this test reveals obstructions in the spinal cord.
- Describe likely adverse effects from injection of contrast medium, including a transient burning sensation, a flushed feeling, transient headache, nausea, or vomiting.
- Explain that the patient may feel some pain during positioning, needle insertion, and, in some cases, removal of the contrast medium.

- Tell the patient that this test helps to determine the presence of fractures, tumors, and other conditions.
- Explain to the patient that his head will be immobilized and that several X-rays of his skull will be taken from various angles.

Test	Pretest care
Vertebral radiography	• No food or fluid restrictions are required. • Have the patient remove all jewelry, metal objects, and other items that might obscure anatomic detail in the films.
Cerebral angiography	• Restrict food and fluid for 8 to 10 hours before the test. • Administer a sedative and an anticholinergic drug 30 to 45 minutes before the test, if ordered. • Note hypersensitivity to contrast medium on the patient's chart. • Have the patient put on a hospital gown and remove all jewelry, dentures, hairpins, and other objects that may obscure anatomic details.

Posttest care	Patient instruction
• No post-test care is required.	• Explain that this test permits examination of the spine. • Advise the patient that he will be placed in various positions during the examination. • Tell him to remain as still as possible and to hold his breath when asked.
• Observe for bleeding, check distal pulses, and apply a pressure bandage to the puncture site. • Maintain bedrest for 12 to 24 hours. • Administer pain medications as prescribed. • Monitor vital signs and neurologic status for 24 hours. • Observe the puncture site for signs of extravasation. Apply an ice bag to reduce discomfort and minimize swelling. If bleeding occurs, apply pressure to the puncture site. • After a femoral approach, keep the affected leg straight for 12 hours, and routinely check distal pulses; monitor temperature, color, and sensation of the affected limb with each vital-sign check. • After a carotid artery approach, monitor for dysphagia and respiratory distress. • Also monitor for disorientation and weakness or numbness in the extremities and observe for arterial spasms, which may produce symptoms of transient ischemic attacks. • After a brachial approach, immobilize the affected arm for 6 hours or longer and frequently check the radial pulse. If the hand or arm becomes pale, cool, or numb, report the changes immediately. • Use a sign to warn personnel not to take blood pressures in the affected arm. • Encourage drinking fluids to flush out the dye. • Resume the patient's usual diet.	• Explain that this test assesses blood circulation in the brain. • Tell the patient that he will be positioned on an X-ray table with his head immobilized and that he should remain still when asked. • Describe possible adverse effects of contrast medium, such as a transient burning sensation as the medium is injected, a warm flushed feeling, transient headache, a salty taste, or nausea or vomiting after the dye is injected.

Selected references

Clinical Laboratory Tests: Values and Implications. Springhouse, Pa.: Springhouse Corp., 1991.

Diseases. Springhouse, Pa.: Springhouse Corp., 1993.

Gorssman, R.I., and Yousen, D.M. *Neuroradiology: The Requisites.* St. Louis: Mosby–Year Book, Inc., 1993.

Handbook of Medical-Surgical Nursing. Springhouse, Pa.: Springhouse Corp., 1994.

Illustrated Guide to Diagnostic Tests. Springhouse, Pa.: Springhouse Corp., 1996.

Lewis, S.M., and Collier, I.C. *Medical-Surgical Nursing: Assessment and Management of Clinical Problems,* 4th ed. St. Louis: Mosby–Year Book, Inc., 1995.

Marieb, E.N. *Human Anatomy and Physiology,* 3rd ed. Redwood City, Ca.: Benjamin/Cummings Publishing Co., Inc., 1995.

McCance, K.L., and Huether, S.E. *Pathophysiology: The Biological Basis for Disease in Adults and Children,* 2nd ed. St.Louis: Mosby–Year Book, Inc., 1994.

Osborn, A. G. *Diagnostic Neuroradiology.* St. Louis: Mosby–Year Book, Inc., 1994.

Professional Handbook of Diagnostic Tests. Springhouse, Pa.: Springhouse Corp., 1995.

Taveras, J.M., and Ferrucci, J.T. *Radiology: Diagnosis-Imaging-Intervention, vol. 4.* Philadelphia: J.B. Lippincott Co., 1996.

8 Musculoskeletal system

The musculoskeletal system is a network of muscles and bones that give the body form and, along with an intricate system of tendons, ligaments, joints, allow it to maneuver. The musculoskeletal system also protects the body's organs and produces red blood cells in the marrow that fills the inside of long and large bones. Bones are made of inorganic minerals and salts, such as calcium and phosphate, embedded in a framework of collagen fibers.

Anatomy

The anatomy of the musculoskeletal system includes muscles and bones and the structures that surround and support them.

Muscles

The body has three major muscle types: skeletal (voluntary, striated), visceral (involuntary, smooth), and cardiac. Viewed through a microscope, skeletal muscle appears as long bands, or striations. (See *Inside a muscle*, page 330.) Skeletal muscle functions voluntarily; contraction can be controlled at will. Exercise, nutrition, gender, and genetic factors account for muscle strength and size.

Tendons

These bands of fibrous connective tissue attach muscle to the periosteum, the double-layered, fibrous membrane covering the bone. Tendons enable bones to move when skeletal muscles contract.

Inside a muscle

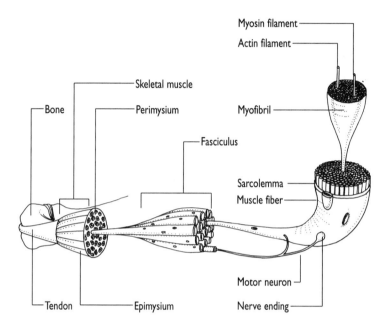

Ligaments

Dense, strong, flexible bands of fibrous connective tissue, ligaments attach one bone to another. Ligaments of concern in a musculoskeletal assessment are those that connect the joint ends (articular ends) of the bones. These ligaments either limit or facilitate movement and provide structural integrity.

Bones

Eighty bones form the axial skeleton, which consists of the head and trunk. Among the structures of the axial skeleton are the skull, facial bones, spine, vertebrae, ribs, and sternum. The appendicular skeleton has 126 bones that compose the arms, legs, shoulder, and pelvic girdles.

Classified by shape and location, bones may be long (humerus, radius, femur, and tibia), short (carpals and tarsals), flat (scapula, ribs, and skull), irregular (vertebrae and mandi-

Inside a bone

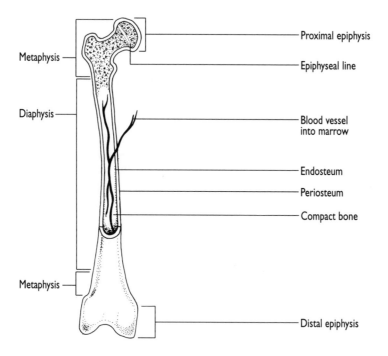

Proximal epiphysis

Metaphysis

Epiphyseal line

Diaphysis

Blood vessel
into marrow

Endosteum

Periosteum

Compact bone

Metaphysis

Distal epiphysis

ble), or sesamoid (patella). Bone tissue is of two basic types: compact and spongy (cancellous). Compact bone is dense and looks smooth and uniform. Spongy bone is composed of small needlelike or flat pieces of bone called trabeculae. Spongy bone has large amounts of open space.

The long axis of a bone, called the shaft or diaphysis, is made of a thick collar of compact bone that surrounds a medullary cavity. In adults, the medullary cavity contains fat (yellow marrow) and is called the yellow bone marrow cavity. This long shaft merges into a broader, neck-like portion called the metaphysis, composed of spongy bone. The end of the bone, the epiphysis, has a thin layer of compact bone on the outside and red marrow on the inside. In young bones, cartilage at the end of the shaft, where the metaphysis and the epiphysis meet, allows space for the long bone to lengthen as the body grows. (See *Inside a bone,* page 331.)

The periosteum helps protect the bone. The outer layer of the periosteum is made of dense, irregular connective tissue; the inner layer, abutting the bone surface, consists primarily of bone-forming cells, or osteoblasts. The periosteum is densely laced with nerve fibers, lymphatic vessels, and blood vessels, which enter the bone through the nutrient foramina. The nutrient foramina is secured to the bone by tufts of collagen called Sharpey's fibers. Tendons and ligaments anchor at the periosteum and Sharpey's fibers are very dense at these junctions of tendons, ligaments, and bones. An exception to the covering on epiphyseal surfaces is found at the junction of long bones that articulate, or move. There, the bones are covered with a smooth articular cartilage that cushions the bone ends and absorbs stress during joint movement.

The spongy bone of the medullary cavity is lined with a thin membrane called the endosteum. Flat bones, on the other hand, consist of two thin plates of compact bone separated by spongy bone called the diploë. Surfaces of flat bone are covered with periosteum, and endosteum lines the inner portion of the bone that contains the marrow.

Cartilage

Cartilage is a dense, connective tissue made of fibers embedded in a strong, gel-like substance. Cartilage is avascular and has no nerve endings.

Cartilage may be fibrous, hyaline, or elastic. Fibrous cartilage forms the symphysis pubis and the intervertebral disks. Hyaline cartilage covers the articular bone surfaces, where one or more bones meet at a joint. Hyaline cartilage also connects the ribs to the sternum and appears in the trachea, bronchi, and nasal septum. Elastic cartilage is located in the auditory canal and the intervertebral disks. It also cushions and absorbs shock, preventing direct transmission of force to the bone.

Joints

The junction of two or more bones is a joint. Major joints are classified by extent of movement.

Synarthrodial joints, such as the cranial sutures, permit no movement. This type of joint has a thin layer of fibrous connective tissue separating the bones. These are also called fibrous joints.

Amphiarthrodial joints, such as the symphysis pubis, allow slight movement. Hyaline cartilage separates the bone in this kind of joint. These are also called cartilaginous joints.

Diarthrodial joints, such as the ankle, wrist, knee, hip, and shoulder, permit free movement. These are also called synovial joints. Separating the bones that form a diarthrodial joint is a cavity lined by a synovial membrane that secretes a viscous lubricating substance called synovial fluid. The membrane is encased in a fibrous joint capsule. This capsule — along with ligaments, tendons, and muscles — helps to stabilize the joint.

Shape and motion are other criteria used to further classify joints, such as ball-and-socket, hinge, and pivot joints.

Bursae

Located at friction points and around joints between tendons, ligaments, and bones, bursae — small synovial sacs — act as cushions to decrease stress on adjacent structures. Bursae, for instance, include the shoulder's subacromial bursa and the knee's prepatellar bursa.

Imaging techniques

Several techniques are used to study the musculoskeletal system. Each requires specific patient care. (For details, see *Guide to patient care*, pages 358 to 361.)

• Plain X-rays are the most common initial screening technique and the most useful diagnostic tool for evaluating structural or functional changes in musculoskeletal diseases. X-rays obtained in multiple views, for example, will reveal most dislocations and fractures. They are also the main technique for detecting and monitoring scoliosis.

• Computed tomography (CT) scanning is more sensitive than plain X-rays to most bone abnormalities. It's useful in imaging bone conditions, such as malignant tumors, that may affect surrounding tissues and for identifying calcium deposits and guiding percutaneous bone biopsy.

• Magnetic resonance imaging (MRI) can detect problems with the spine and spinal cord, and can identify articular abnormalities in soft tissue. Its axial, coronal, and sagittal images aid detection of tendon and ligament disruption. It doesn't use ionizing radiation and is highly sensitive to malignant bone tumors.

• Myelography, an invasive procedure, evaluates abnormalities of the spinal canal and cord. It entails injection of a radiopaque contrast medium into the subarachnoid space.

• Arthrography involves injection of contrast medium to show the shape and integrity of a joint capsule. It has been largely replaced by the noninvasive, more accurate MRI.

• Arthroscopy is the visual examination of a joint interior with a fiber-optic endoscope.

• Nuclear medicine bone scans identify a variety of musculoskeletal conditions. They are a good way of surveying the entire skeleton with relatively low doses of radiation. Nuclear scans are also excellent for detecting bone and joint inflammatory processes. Stress fractures, which may not be detected on plain X-rays, are usually seen clearly on bone scans, which are also good at showing metastatic bone tumors.

Pathophysiology

Many conditions — inflammatory, congenital, or degenerative — may affect the function and movement of the musculoskeletal system.

Inflammatory disorders

Inflammatory disorders may invade bones or joints, creating pain and limiting mobility. These conditions may be acute or chronic. They include rheumatoid arthritis, tendinitis, bursitis, and osteomyelitis.

Rheumatoid arthritis

This autoimmune disease affects connective tissue, causing it to inflame. It primarily affects the small joints of the hands, wrists, and feet and is three times more prevalent in females than males. The cause of rheumatoid arthritis is unknown, but it is believed to affect people who are genetically susceptible. Theories suggest an aberrant immune response to bacteria, mycoplasmas, or viral antigens.

The immune response causes production of self-destructive autoantibodies, called rheumatoid factors (RFs). RFs are usually found in the serum and synovial membranes of patients with rheumatoid arthritis and signal an inflammatory response that leads to synovitis. As the response spreads to surrounding tissues, edema and erosion of the synovial membrane lead to erosion and deterioration of the articular cartilage. In an attempt to heal itself, the synovial membrane releases fibrin to the denuded areas and granulation tissue called pannus forms. Regeneration doesn't occur and the pannus develops into scar tissue that may extend into the joint capsule and bone, causing destruction. In advanced rheumatoid arthritis, the bone atrophies and the joint becomes malaligned, deformed, and fused, resulting in fibrous ankylosis.

⇨ Clinical signs

Onset of rheumatoid arthritis is insidious, beginning with systemic fatigue, weakness, anorexia, weight loss, and a generalized achiness and stiffness. Localization of symptoms occurs gradually with joints becoming painful, tender, and stiff. Early pain is from associated edema and pressure. When palpated, the joint may feel boggy. Skin over the affected joint may by cyanotic, thin, and shiny.

As the disease progresses, joint mobility decreases and deformities, such nodules of fibrinoid and cellular debris, may occur in up to 20% of patients. These deformities are most common in subcutaneous tissue over the extensor surfaces of elbows and fingers. Nodules may be movable or fixed to tendons or bone, and may occur elsewhere in the body. Blood analysis usually shows elevated RF and sedimentation rate values.

Radiographic findings

Plain X-rays reveal:
* loss of joint space and cartilage, periarticular bone erosion, and joint subluxation (see *Rheumatoid arthritis of the hands*)
* soft tissue swelling (frequently an early finding)
* bones appearing as osteoporotic and more radiolucent before erosion can be seen, with malalignment of the affected joints often apparent as the disease progresses
* joint fusion, in advanced disease.

Treatment

Conservative treatment is usually pursued, with surgery reserved for advanced disease. Conservative therapy includes resting the inflamed joint and the body for several hours daily. Hot or cold packs, physical therapy, antineoplastic drugs, a diet high in calories and vitamins, and anti-inflammatory drugs taken orally or injected into the joint may all be used.

Surgical synovectomy may be done early in the disease to remove pannus and decrease inflammatory effusion. Joint realignment or replacement may be used to correct malalignment and deformity and restore mobility.

Tendinitis and bursitis

Inflammation of the tendons (tendinitis) may be caused by acute trauma or by wear and tear from work or sports. Other causes include infection, inflammatory processes like rheumatoid arthritis, crystal-deposition diseases like gout, abnormalities of bony alignment, and hypermobility in a joint.

Chronic inflammation of a tendon may lead to degeneration and tears. The most common sites are the Achilles tendon and the muscles and tendons of the shoulder. With chronic irritation, calcification may lead to calcific tendinitis.

Bursitis involves inflammation of the bursa from repeated

Rheumatoid arthritis of the hands

This plain X-ray of the hands of a 43-year-old man with a long history of arthitis show classic signs of rheumatoid arthritis. Note the periarticular soft tissue swelling ⇒ and many erosions involving the distal ulna, carpals, metacarpals, and phalanges ⇾. Narrowing of the joint spaces is also apparent. Also note the periarticular osteoporosis around the metacarpal and phalangeal joints ✱.

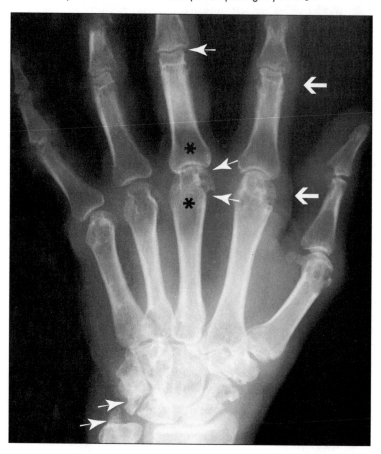

joint trauma or other stress. It usually affects middle-aged people. The shoulder is the most common site, but bursitis may also occur in the knees, elbows, or hips. Associated inflammatory joint diseases may also cause it. Septic bursitis is caused by bacterial infection of a wound or the skin over the bursa. Calcium may invade the bursa, worsening the condition.

⮞ Clinical signs

Pain and local inflammation are the initial symptoms in both conditions. Limited movement because of increasing pain is also seen. The skin over the inflamed region may be warm to the touch. Edema may be present.

⮞ Radiographic findings

MRI is used to view tendon abnormalities. The following findings may be seen in the disorders listed.

Tendinitis
   • focal or diffuse swelling and heterogeneity of the tendon
   • well-demonstrated presence of excessive fluid in the tendon sheath (tenosynovitis), appearing as a well-circumscribed halo of fluid around the tendon
   • tear showing disruption in the continuity of the tendon sheath. (See *Rotator cuff tear.*)
   Plain X-rays and CT scans may show calcium deposits as speckled, radiopaque densities following the position of the tendon.

Bursitis
   • calcified, radiopaque densities around the bursa seen on plain X-rays or CT scans (most common at the shoulder).

⮞ Treatment

Tendinitis is treated conservatively with cold packs, anti-inflammatories (both oral or injected into the inflamed tendon), and analgesics. Rest and immobilization usually bring symptomatic relief.

Rotator cuff tear

This coronal-plane MRI scan in figure A reveals a tear of the right rotator cuff ➔. The 60-year-old woman complained of right shoulder pain and inability to move her shoulder freely. In figure B the saggital MRI image of the knee of a 35 year old male injured while skiing reveals an oblique tear ➔ in the posterior horn of the medial meniscus.

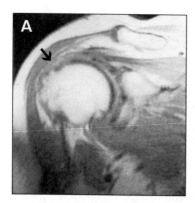

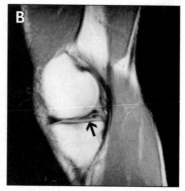

Bursitis is treated conservatively at first with immobilization of the affected joint. Analgesics and anti-inflammatories are used. Warm moist heat is usually applied for temporary relief. Injection of steroids into the affected area may be needed if conservative therapy fails to bring relief.

Osteomyelitis

This is a bone infection usually caused by the bacterium *Staphylococcus aureus.* Other sources of infection may be fungal, parasitic, and viral. The infection may be chronic or acute. Osteomyelitis is classified by mode of transmission as hematogenous or exogenous. Hematogenous osteomyelitis is caused by blood-borne pathogens. Infection may spread from the bone to the surrounding adjacent soft tissues.

Exogenous osteomyelitis may be caused by contamination from bacteria in superficial wounds that spread to the bone. The condition may also be caused by human or animal bites that allow bacteria in superficial wounds to migrate to the bone. Deep, penetrating bites may infect the bone directly.

Direct bone contamination can also occur from open fractures or dislocations with skin laceration. Other iatrogenic causes are orthopedic surgery, prosthetic insertion, I.V. punctures, and I.M. and intra-articular injections.

The infection causes the bone to weaken, deteriorate, and undergo other changes, such as disruption of the cortex, which can make the bone susceptible to fractures.

⇨ Clinical signs

Acute hematogenous osteomyelitis causes abrupt inflammation. Redness, heat, pain, and edema may be present. Systemic symptoms of fever, malaise, fatigue, chills, nausea, anorexia, and weight loss may occur. The condition may progress from acute to subacute to chronic if not effectively treated.

Exogenous osteomyelitis usually exhibits symptoms of soft-tissue infection. Exudate may disrupt muscles and supporting tissues, and form abscesses. Fever, lymphadenopathy, local pain, and swelling usually occur within days of the initial cause. Mobility of the affected area is limited.

⇨ Radiographic findings

It may be 10 to 14 days before radiographic findings of osteomyelitis can be detected. Such findings may mimic those of other disorders.

The following plain X-ray findings indicate bone infection:
• erosions
• aggressive bone destruction
• periostitis
• soft-tissue swelling
• osteosclerosis (chalky or opaque appearance with obliteration of distinct borders between cortex and trabeculae)
• bone fragmentation
• fractures
• subluxation

• ill-defined bone contours.

Bone scans are usually done early because the infection site may be detected within 48 hours of symptom onset, many days before other radiographic findings are apparent.

A bone scan may reveal:

• *hot spots*, areas where the bone absorbs more radioisotope than other areas

• greater radioisotope absorption in the infected areas because of increased blood flow and metabolism of bone at the infection site. (See *Osteomyelitis of the foot*, page 342.)

⇨ Treatment

Treatment includes aggressive I.V. antibiotic therapy after the infecting organism is identified. A percutaneous needle aspiration under radiographic guidance may be needed to collect the specimen. The site may be drained surgically to relieve pressure and to remove sequestrum. Usually, the infected bone is immobilized with a cast or traction, or by complete bed rest. The patient receives analgesics and I.V. fluids as needed.

If an abscess forms, treatment includes incision and drainage, followed by a culture of the drainage. Anti-infective therapy may include systemic antibiotics, intracavitary instillation of antibiotics, or local application of packed, wet, antibiotic-soaked dressings.

Chronic osteomyelitis may require surgery, such as sequestrectomy to remove dead bone and saucerization to promote drainage and decrease pressure.

Degenerative conditions

Degenerative conditions, such as osteoarthritis and degenerative disk disease, may be caused by aging or may develop from continued wear and tear. These conditions are classified as inflammatory or noninflammatory.

Osteoarthritis

Osteoarthritis is the most common type of arthritis. It causes deterioration of the joint cartilage and formation of reactive

Osteomyelitis of the foot

This bone scan of a 62-year-old woman with fever and a swollen, red right foot reveals a *"hot spot"* area of increased activity in the middle foot ◊ consistent with osteomyelitis. Activity in the great toe → results from degenerative arthritis.

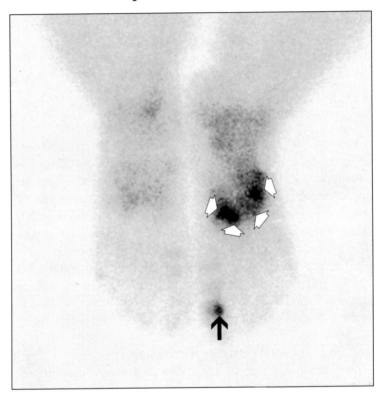

new bone at the margins and subchondral areas of the joints. This chronic degeneration results from a breakdown of cartilage, most often in the hips and knees.

Osteoarthritis is classified as primary (idiopathic) or secondary (related to a specific event or condition). Joints of the hands, knees, and hips are most often affected. As the cartilage degenerates, fibrillation, or fissure formation, occurs and further thins the cartilage. The underlying bone is unprotected, causing it to become dense and hard. Cysts may develop in the bone ends and communicate with the joint through the cartilage fissures. Bony projections known as osteophytes may form under the degenerated cartilage. The degenerative process leads to inflammation of the synovium and the joint effusion and bone erosion that follow synovial inflammation.

⇨ Clinical signs

Joint pain is the overriding symptom of osteoarthritis. It's aggravated by use and relieved with rest. Other common symptoms include stiffness, limited range of motion (ROM), swelling, muscle wasting, instability, partial dislocation, and deformity. Limitations in mobility are caused by muscle spasm, capsular scarring, and deformity of the joints. Frequently, the movement of the joint produces a sound of crepitus, creaking, or grating.

⇨ Radiographic findings

Plain X-rays are often taken to assess osteoarthritis. Findings include:
* joint narrowing and bone sclerosis (see *Osteoarthritis of the knee,* page 345)
* presence of osteophytes, bony overgrowths that give the bone a lumpy or irregular contour, a hallmark of osteoarthritis
* cyst-like lesions in the subarticular area, which appear as small, radiolucent, circular or piriform areas that may extend to the joint surface.

Bone scans can survey all potentially arthritic sites with one exam. They are better at depicting diseased joints than plain X-rays are, especially when a contrast medium is used. Areas of increased tracer uptake may denote arthritic or degenerative conditions.

⇨ Treatment

Treatment is mainly palliative; degenerative joint disease is a progressive disease without cure. Analgesics, moist heat, ROM exercises, anti-inflammatories, frequent rest periods, and use of a cane or crutches to avoid bearing weight on the affected joints may temporarily relieve symptoms. Surgery to repair or correct deformities or replace diseased joints is used in severe cases.

Degenerative disk disease
Degeneration of the intervertebral disks is a common effect of aging and affects almost everyone older than age 60 to some degree. The condition is prevalent in men, especially men who have done heavy physical labor for extended periods.

Degenerative disk disease may also be a manifestation of osteoarthritis. Early changes from the disease are related to degeneration and dehydration of the disk in which the disk space narrows. The stress promotes osteophyte formation. As the disk continues weakening, its nucleus may protrude and the protruding fragment may crowd the spinal canal and compress the cord or nerve roots.

⇨ Clinical signs

Degenerative disk disease is usually asymptomatic until the apophyseal, uncovertebral, or costovertebral, joints are affected. Mild aching and stiffness occur first, followed by more severe and chronic back pain. If nerve roots are compressed, the pain may radiate and sensory and motor function may be affected.

⇨ Radiographic findings

Plain X-ray studies of the spine are essential to show degenerative changes and to rule out other abnormalities. Films may not show a herniated disk because even marked disk prolapse may show up as normal.

The following findings may occur:
- osteophytes on the anterior and posterior vertebral margins
- narrowed disk spaces

Osteoarthritis of the knee

This plain X-ray of a 64-year-old man with pain in his right knee shows medial joint-space narrowing ➔ and mild osteophyte formation ➤.

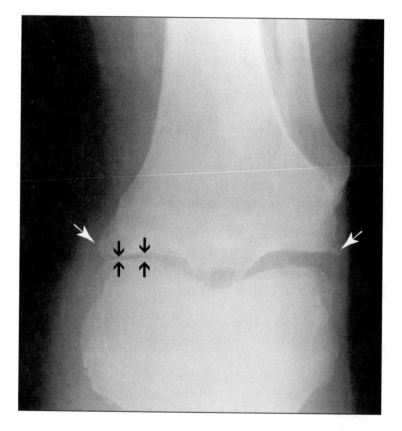

- sclerotic vertebral body end plates
- Schmorl's nodules — from prolapse of the disk into the vertebra — appearing as lucent areas with sclerotic margins in the vertebrae, usually abutting the end plate.

A CT scan reveals the same findings but will also show:
- soft tissue density of the bulging or herniated disk
- any compromise of the nerve roots or spinal cord.

MRI provides similar information and has the advantage of

being able to produce images in the sagittal or coronal planes. Myelography pinpoints herniation level.

⟹ Treatment

Conservative treatment is usually the first line of treatment. Anti-inflammatory drugs, taken orally or injected into the affected site, may bring temporary relief. Bed rest, moist heat, physical therapy, and analgesics may alleviate symptoms. Surgery is reserved for severe cases, usually to relieve nerve-root or spinal-cord compression and to treat instability.

Skeletal tumors

Many different kinds of tumors invade the skeleton. Skeletal tumors may be primary, arising from cells in the musculo-skeletal system, or metastatic, spreading to bones from other primary sites.

Primary skeletal tumors are of four potential cell types: osteogenic (bone cells), chondrogenic (cartilage), collagenic (fibrous tissue), myelogenic (vascular or marrow tissue). Of all primary bone tumor types, multiple myeloma and osteosarco-ma are the most common. Whether the bone tumors are benign or malignant, they may lead to bone destruction, ero-sion or expansion of the cortex, reactive periosteal changes, fractures, and invasion of adjacent soft tissue structures.

Myeloma is the abnormal proliferation of immunocytes (plasma cells) in the bone marrow. It is the most common form of bone cancer, accounting for about 25% of all bone tumors. It may be focal — plasma cytoma — or multifocal — multiple myeloma. It commonly affects people older than age 40 and afflicts men twice as often as women and blacks more often than whites.

Osteosarcoma is a malignant bone tumor. This cancer is the most common primary bone tumor, accounting for 20% of malignant bone neoplasms. It occurs twice as often in men as in women and appears most often in adolescents. Osteo-sarcoma usually occurs in the metaphyseal portion of major tubular bones and metastasizes early, often to the lung.

Any malignancy may metastasize to bone, but the usual primary types metastasize to cause bone, breast, prostate, kidney, thyroid, and lung tumors. Frequent sites of metastatic involvement are the bones that produce red marrow, such as the spine, pelvis, ribs, skull, and the upper ends of the humerus and femur.

Clinical signs

Pain — focally or in the entire skeleton — weakness, fatigue, weight loss, and anorexia are symptoms of myeloma. Initially, the pain is an ache; it's intermittent and aggravated by bearing weight. Severity of the pain progresses as the disease spreads. Usual sites of pain include the lumbar and thoracic regions, the pelvis, the ribs, and the sternum. Often, a patient's condition is treated as arthritis or a ruptured disk until diagnosis is made. Accompanying anemia may produce pallor.

Osteosarcoma also presents with pain at the involvement site. At first, the pain is mild and intermittent but gradually intensifies. Swelling may be present. Blood levels of serum alkaline phosphatase may be elevated.

Metastatic bone lesions may be asymptomatic or produce pain. Pathologic fractures may occur through diseased bone. Serum acid phosphatase levels may be elevated when prostatic metastases are present.

Radiographic findings

Myeloma usually features three X-ray findings, including:
- osteopenia, or a scarcity of bone substance, which appears as bone more radiolucent than normal
- lytic lesions, which may appear as radiolucent, "punched out" areas of bone destruction
- pathologic fractures, which are common in the ribs and vertebrae.

Osteosarcoma may show itself on plain X-rays as:
- an area of destroyed bone that appears to have been eaten by moths

Bone tumor

This plain X-ray shows a well-defined, eccentric, *bubbly* expansile lesion ◊ in the distal femoral diaphysis in a 19-year-old woman with pain in her right thigh.

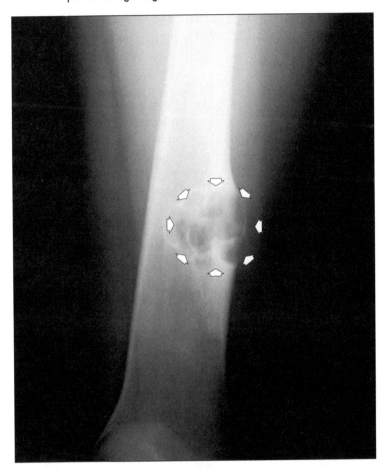

- indistinct borders merging into normal tissue
- abundant periosteal reaction appearing as irregular new bone growth on bone edges. (See *Bone tumor.*)

Metastatic lesions often involve red marrow sites, such as the spine, pelvis, ribs, skull, and the upper ends of the humerus and the femur. These lesions are usually osteolytic (with destruction of bone tissue) or osteosclerotic (with increased density in the affected bone). Osteolytic lesions present the following findings on plain X-rays:

• ragged, irregular defects in the bone that are mottled or radiolucent

• no sclerosis along the margin, with the periosteum seldom involved.

Osteosclerotic type lesions appear on plain X-rays as:

• foci of dense areas or as a diffuse density involving a large area in the bone. A mixed type of metastasis that appears to be bone sclerosis and destruction may also be present. The affected bone will appear mottled with areas of lysis and sclerosis.

Nuclear bone scans will usually show:

• metastases as areas of increased uptake of the radionuclide. Bone scans are often used to survey the entire body after a primary tumor is identified to check for bone involvement. Lesions are often detected on bone scans when plain X-rays appear normal. Bone scans are also used to see how the bone metastasis is responding to therapy.

CT scanning and MRI may be used to detect and stage metastatic tumors of the bone. Both are more sensitive than plain X-rays. MRI is the most accurate imaging technique for detection of metastases.

⇨ Treatment

Treatment of multiple myeloma includes narcotics and pressure-reducing beds to help alleviate discomfort. Chemotherapy is used to treat diffuse disease. Radiation therapy may be used for focused bone-lesion treatment.

Treatment of osteosarcoma usually involves amputation of the affected bone. Chemotherapy may improve survival chances if the disease is discovered before metastasis. Radiation therapy is also used to help arrest the disease. Osteosarcoma is usually fatal within two years of discovery.

Trauma

Trauma — blunt, sharp, or forceful — can result in a variety of injuries to the musculoskeletal system, causing symptoms ranging from minor pain to severe complications. Each year, 1 of 10 people sustains a musculoskeletal injury. The most common of these injuries are fractures, dislocations, sprains, and strains.

Fractures

As soon as bones are fractured, they begin repairing themselves. The healing process has four phases: hematoma formation, fibrocartilaginous callus formation, bony callus formation, and remodeling.

In most cases, fractures are accompanied by hemorrhage from broken blood vessels in the bone, periosteum, and surrounding tissue. A hematoma forms at the fracture site and bone cells deprived of nutrition begin to die.

The speed at which bones heal depends on many factors, including severity of injury, type and amount of bone tissue damaged, blood supply, patient age, treatment, complications, and severity and type of other pathologic conditions.

Fractures are classified as complete, incomplete, compound, or simple. In a complete fracture, a bone is broken through; in an incomplete fracture, the bone may be only partially broken. In so-called simple fractures, bone fragments don't penetrate the skin; in compound fractures, they do penetrate. Fractures may also be classified by the direction of the fracture line, location of the fracture, or degree of malalignment.

⟜ Clinical signs

Clinical signs vary according to type and location of fractures. General signs and symptoms include deformity, swelling, pain, tenderness, muscle spasm, impaired sensation, and limited ROM and extreme pain on movement of the bone.

Leg fractures

Figure A is an anteroposterior X-ray projection of the left leg and ankle of a 21-year-old man who was involved in a motorcycle accident. Note the oblique, comminuted fracture of the tibia ➔ with lateral displacement of distal parts. Note also a comminuted avulsion type fracture of the medial malleolus ➤. Figure B is a CT scan done on a 38-year-old woman who fell off a ladder. The axial image through the distal femur and knee joint shows a linear, minimally displaced fracture ➔ of the lateral condyle extending into the joint. Note joint effusion ✳ and the patella **P**.

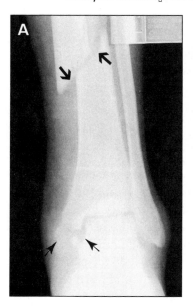

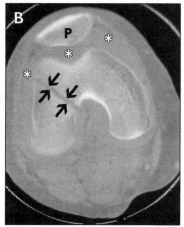

➥ Radiographic findings

Plain X-rays are the first imaging technique used to find suspected fractures. Two views are needed — one to see the fracture and one to assess angulation and displacement. The films show:

- displacement of bone fragments
- radiolucent breaks in bone continuity
- malalignment of joints

• associated soft tissue edema. (See *Leg fractures*, page 351.)
Bone scans may reveal stress fractures or subtle fractures
that may not show up on plain X-rays. The scans will show:
• an increase in tracer uptake in the area of fracture, usually
within 24 to 48 hours.

Arthrograms may detect and confirm suspected tendon or
ligament damage in joint trauma. The contrast dye injected
into the joint cavity may show:
• a disruption in the continuity of the torn structure.

CT scanning is reserved for complicated fractures or for
fractures that are difficult to diagnose.

MRI may show fractures that other techniques can't. It's
particularly useful in assessing damage and extent of injuries
before bone scans or X-rays show the fracture and in detecting
damage to cartilage, ligaments, tendons, and surrounding soft
tissue.

➥ Treatment

Treatment of fractures centers on realigning the bone and
immobilizing the bone and fragments of it until the bone can
heal itself. Surgical and nonsurgical techniques are used to
reduce fractures. Splints, casts, traction, and other external fixation devices may be used to nonsurgically immobilize fractured bones. Surgical procedures may include the placement of
pins, plates, and screws for internal fixation of fractured bones.

Dislocations

Dislocations refer to displacement or malalignment of two
bones. Subluxation refers to partial loss of contact between
two bones. Joints most often affected by dislocation and subluxation include the knee, shoulder, elbow, wrist, finger, and
hip.

Dislocations may occur anteriorly, posteriorly, superiorly, or
inferiorly, depending on the direction of the force that caused
the injury. In dislocations, the bone is damaged and adjacent
structures, including the nerves, blood vessels, ligaments, ten-

dons, and other soft tissue, may become bruised or torn.

↪ Clinical signs

Signs of a dislocation include swelling, abnormal alignment, pain, limitation of movement, and joint deformity.

↪ Radiographic findings

Plain X-rays confirm the diagnosis and identify any associated fractures. They may reveal:
* malaligned bones
* subluxation
* cracks, avulsions, or breaks marking associated fractures.

↪ Treatment

Treatment for a dislocation includes immediate reduction (before tissue edema and muscle spasm make reduction difficult) to prevent additional tissue damage and vascular impairment. (See "Case study: Hit-and-run accident victim with knee dislocation," page 355.)

Closed reduction consists of manual traction. Open reduction may include wire fixation of the joint, skeletal traction, and ligament repair. After reduction, a splint, a cast, or traction immobilizes the joint.

Sprains and strains

Sprains and strains are usually less severe than fractures or dislocations but can also produce intense pain and may disable a person. A sprain is a complete or incomplete tear in the supporting ligaments surrounding a joint. It may cause an avulsion fracture, which occurs when a bone fragment is pulled out of place by a ligament.

A strain is an injury to a muscle or tendinous attachment. An injury to a tendon or ligament may lead to instability and pain and eventually cause acute or chronic dislocation or subluxation. A chronic strain results from the accumulated effects of repeated muscle overuse.

⮑ Clinical signs

Swelling is a key sign of a sprain. A sprain causes local pain that worsens during joint movement. Usually, mobility is limited or lost, but it's typically not affected until several hours after the sprain occurs. Examination will reveal ecchymosis from blood extravasating into surrounding tissue. In a moderate or severe sprain, palpation may reveal point tenderness.

A strain reveals swelling over the injury site and, if the injury is several days old, ecchymosis. Palpation reveals the degree of swelling and defines the area of tenderness. An acute strain may cause sharp, transient pain and rapid swelling. When the severe pain has subsided, the patient may complain of muscle tenderness. There may be a snapping or popping noise at the site of the injury. Patients with chronic strain will report stiffness, soreness, and generalized tenderness.

⮑ Radiographic findings

Plain X-rays rule out fractures and confirm ligament damage.

⮑ Treatment

In either type of injury, ice should be applied to the site immediately to control swelling. After 24 to 48 hours, treatment should switch to heat to encourage reabsorption of blood and to promote healing and comfort.

The patient may need surgery if the muscle, tendon, or ligament ruptures or if the ligaments torn by a sprain don't heal properly and cause a recurrent dislocation. A rehabilitation or exercise program may help ensure a gradual progressive resumption of activity.

Case study: Hit-and-run accident victim with knee dislocation

While walking to work one morning, Mr. Sitton was struck by a hit-and-run driver. The impact threw him about 20 feet. He landed on his left leg. When he arrived by ambulance at the hospital, Mr. Sitton had stable vital signs, a cervical collar was in place, and I.V. access had been obtained. He complained

Angiogram of knee

This angiogram shows posterior bowing of the popliteal artery ⇒ caused by swelling and joint effusion.

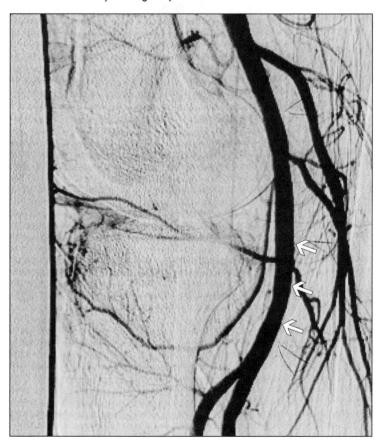

Knee damage in MRI scans

The sagittal MRI scan in figure A reveals a rupture of the anterior cruciate ligament ⇒ and bucking of the posterior cruciate →➤ that caused avulsion of the ligament at the time of knee dislocation. Note the hemorrhagic knee effusion ➡. The coronal MRI scan in figure B shows a subchondral fracture of the lateral femoral condyl ➡ and a subtle, subchondral lateral tibial plateau fracture →➤.

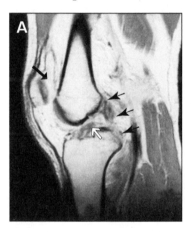
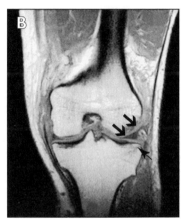

mainly of soreness in the thoracic region of his back and extreme pain in his left leg.

An examination revealed an obvious external-rotation dislocation of the left knee, with possible fracture. Distal pulses were strong but sensation in the left foot was diminished.

X-rays of the spine, left leg, and knee were ordered to assess damage. No fractures or dislocations were seen in the spine. The knee and leg, however, showed an anterior-lateral dislocation of the tibia under the femur.

In the emergency department, the orthopedic surgeon advised a closed reduction after reviewing the films with the radiologist. Mr. Sitton was given 4 mg of morphine sulphate by I.V. push, and closed reduction of the knee was performed. An immobilizer was placed on his leg and ice and elevation ordered. After the reduction, the orthopedic surgeon was concerned about vascular supply to the knee because of the extent of the injuries, and an arteriogram was ordered.

The arteriogram revealed that the arteries supplying the knee were intact, though displaced by the dislocation. (See *Angiogram of knee*, page 355.)

Mr. Sitton, however, continued to complain of decreased sensation in the foot. An MRI scan revealed a tear in the anterior cruciate, medial, and posterior collateral ligaments. The menisci and patellar tendon were intact. The scan also revealed injury to the lateral femoral condyle, lateral tibial plateau, and a large joint effusion. (See *Knee damage in MRI scans.*)

Reconstructive surgery was scheduled for 2 weeks later. In the meantime, Mr. Sitton was discharged and went home 2 days after the accident, with plans for surgery and expectations of a full recovery.

Guide to patient care

This chart lists patient preparation and pretest and posttest care for various diagnostic-imaging tests of the musculoskeletal system.

Test	Pretest care
Skeletal computed tomography	• Restrict food for 4 hours before the test if the use of contrast medium is anticipated. If not, no food or fluid restrictions are required. • Administer a sedative if prescribed. • Note hypersensitivity to contrast medium on the patient's chart. • Have the patient remove any metal objects that might obscure anatomic detail in the scan.
Skeletal magnetic resonance imaging	• No food or fluid restrictions are required. • Administer a sedative as ordered if the patient suffers from claustrophobia. • Have the patient remove all metal objects including jewelry. Also ask if the patient has any surgically implanted metal joints, pins, clips, valves, pumps, or pacemakers that could be attracted by the strong MRI magnet. If he does, he cannot have the test.

Posttest care	Patient instruction
• Resume the patient's usual diet.	• Explain that this test permits visualization of bones and joints. • Inform the patient that he will be positioned on an X-ray table and that the scanner will make loud, clacking sounds as it rotates around his body. • Inform the patient that he may experience transient adverse effects such as a flushed feeling, metallic taste, or headache following injection of contrast medium.
• Observe the patient for postural hypotension if the study takes longer than normal.	• Explain that this test assesses the status of joints, bones, and soft tissues. • Explain that this test is not painful and involves no exposure to radiation from the scanner. Mention that a radioactive contrast medium may be used, depending on the type of tissue being studied. • Ask the patient if he suffers from claustrophobia. If so, he may require sedation. • Tell the patient he will hear the scanner clicking, whirring, and thumping as it moves. • Reassure the patient that he will be able to communicate at all times.

Test	Pretest care
Vertebral radiography	• No food or fluid restrictions are required. • Have the patient remove all jewelry, metal objects, and other objects that might obscure anatomic detail in the X-ray films.
Arthrography	• No food or fluid restrictions are required unless contrast medium is used. In those cases, restrict food and fluid for 4 hours before the test. • Note hypersensitivity to contrast medium on the patient's chart.
Bone scan	• Restrict food and fluid for 4 hours before the test if use of contrast medium is anticipated. • Administer analgesics as ordered for pain. • Note hypersensitivity to contrast medium on the patient's chart. • Have the patient void immediately before the test.

Posttest care	**Patient instruction**
• No posttest care is required.	• Explain that this test permits examination of the spine. • Advise the patient that he will be placed in various positions during the examination. • Inform the patient that he must remain as still as possible and will need to hold his breath when requested.
• If an arthroscope was used to inspect a knee joint, tell the patient to leave the bandage in place for several days. Also show the patient how to rewrap the knee. • Advise the patient to rest the joint for at least 12 hours. • Expect some swelling or discomfort after the test. Crepitant noises may be heard in the joint after the test. Those symptoms usually disappear after 1 or 2 days. • Tell the patient to report persistent symptoms. • Apply ice to the joint if swelling occurs, and administer a mild analgesic as ordered for pain.	• Explain that this test permits examination of joints. • Inform the patient that the fluoroscope allows the doctor to trace the contrast dye as it fills the joint space. • Explain that standard X-ray films may be taken after diffusion of contrast medium. • Inform the patient that even though his joint will be anesthetized, he may experience a tingling sensation or pressure in the joint as the contrast medium is injected. • Advise the patient to cooperate fully and quickly in assuming various positions. The films must be taken as quickly as possible to ensure optimum quality.
• Check the injection site for redness or swelling. If a hematoma develops, apply warm soaks as ordered. • Monitor for residual adverse effects from the injection of contrast medium. • Have the patient increase his fluid intake for 1 to 3 hours after injection of the tracer. The increased fluid intake will facilitate renal clearance of the circulating free tracer.	• Explain that this test can detect abnormal skeletal pathology, often sooner than is possible with ordinary X-ray film. • Advise the patient not to drink large amounts of fluids before the test, since he will need to drink 4 to 6 glasses of water or tea in the interval between injection of the tracer and the actual scanning. Assure the patient that the test is painless. • Ensure that the female patient isn't pregnant.

Selected references

Clinical Laboratory Tests: Values and Implications. Springhouse, Pa.: Springhouse Corp., 1991.

Diseases. Springhouse, Pa.: Springhouse Corporation, 1993.

Laudicina, P.F. *Applied Pathology for Radiographers.* Philadelphia, Pa.: W.B. Saunders Co., 1989.

Lewis, S.M., and Collier, I.C. *Medical-Surgical Nursing: Assessment and Management of Clinical Problems,* 4th ed. St. Louis: Mosby–Year Book, Inc., 1995.

Marieb, E.N. *Human Anatomy and Physiology,* 3rd ed. Redwood City, Ca.: Benjamin/Cummings Publishing Co., Inc., 1995.

McCance, K.L., and Huether, S.E. *Pathophysiology: The Biological Basis for Disease in Adults and Children,* 2nd ed. St. Louis: Mosby–Year Book, Inc., 1994.

Professional Handbook of Diagnostic Tests. Springhouse, Pa.: Springhouse Corp., 1995.

Taveras, J.M., and Ferrucci, J.T. *Radiology: Diagnosing-Imaging-Intervention,* vol. 4. Philadelphia: J.B. Lippincott Co., 1996.

Glossary

Absorption — the taking in of energy, such as ionizing radiation or sound waves, by body tissue or other structures.

Angiography — radiographic examination of one or more arteries after injection of a contrast medium into the femoral artery or, less frequently, the brachial or carotid artery.

Anteroposterior (AP) — from front to back; for example, an AP chest X-ray projection.

Arthrography — radiographic examination of a joint after injection of a radiopaque dye, air, or both to outline soft-tissue structures and joint contour.

Attenuation — loss of energy that occurs as a beam of radiation passes through structures.

Axial — of or pertaining to the axis of a structure; in radiology or ultrasonography, the horizontal cross sections (perpendicular to the axis) in which body parts are imaged.

Cine magnetic resonance imaging (MRI) — computer-assisted imaging technique in which rapid-succession magnetic resonance images are taken and viewed sequentially.

Color-flow Doppler ultrasonography — technique in which color-coded flow direction and velocity information collected by Doppler ultrasonography are superimposed onto a black and white cross-sectional image; using direction (coded as colors) and velocity (coded as shades), the technique produces color maps that show blood flow within the heart chambers.

Compton effect (scatter) — deflection of X-rays unabsorbed by the body and deflected into the environment; causes the rays to lose energy, contributing to a distortion of density on the film and increased radiation exposure to health care personnel.

Computed tomography (CT) — recording of internal body images at a predetermined plane using a tomograph; after a scintillation counter measures the emergent X-ray beam, a computer processes the electronic impulses; cross sections of the body are then reconstructed and displayed.

Cystography — radiographic technique in which X-rays are taken of a bladder filled with contrast medium.

Decubitus — a recumbent position; *dorsal decubitus* refers to a supine position, *ventral decubitus* to a prone position, and *lateral decubitus* to a side-lying position.

Density — degree of darkening on an X-ray film, reflecting the concentration of mass; the denser the mass, the whiter it appears.

Echo — reflection of a sound wave by a surface or an object.

Echogenic focus — in ultrasonography, a concentration of echoes returned to a transducer; for example, gallstones produce an *echogenic focus* because sound waves bounce off them, forming echoes.

Echogenicity — degree to which a structure gives rise to reflections of sound waves, or the property of structures or tissues that reflect sound waves.

Embolization — deliberate occlusion of a blood vessel by catheterization and various mechanical techniques, such as titanium coils, or chemical agents, such as Gelfoam.

Endoscopic retrograde cholangiopancreatography (ERCP) — radiographic examination of the pancreatic ducts and hepatobiliary tree after injection of a contrast medium into the duodenal papilla.

Excretory urography — technique in which contrast medium injected I.V. is filtered by the kidneys and excreted through the ureters and bladder, which are then X-rayed at specific intervals to produce images on film; formerly called intravenous pyelography.

Extracorporeal shock wave lithotripsy (ESWL) — procedure in which a calculus within the gallbladder or urinary system is fragmented using high-intensity sound waves; the fragments are then passed naturally.

Fluoroscopy — radiographic technique that visually examines a part of the body or the function of an organ using a fluoroscope; often yields immediate serial images, which appear on a video monitor.

Gadolinium — chemical compound that, when injected, helps to produce tissue contrast in magnetic resonance imaging scans.

Gamma camera — device that converts photons from a radioactive source within a patient to a light pulse on a screen and subsequently into an image.

Hyperechoic — in ultrasonography, the property of giving off an abundance of echoes compared to adjacent structures; hyperechoic tissues and structures reflect many of the sound waves directed at them.

Hypoechoic — in ultrasonography, the property of giving off few or no echoes compared to adjacent structures; hypoechoic tissues and structures reflect few of the many sound waves directed at them.

Implanted infusion port (implanted access device) — venous infusion system implanted under the patient's skin; consists of a port with a resealable membranous diaphragm connected to a catheter that's threaded into a central vein. The port is accessed externally by puncturing through the skin and the membranous diaphragm with an infusion needle.

Iodinated contrast medium — chemical compound containing iodine that's instilled or injected into or around a body structure to allow radiographic visualization; by blocking the penetration of X-rays, the contrast medium produces a more clearly defined image than is possible with plain imaging.

Ionizing radiation — electromagnetic radiation capable of causing neutral atoms to gain or lose an electron as it passes through matter.

Maximum permissible dose (MPD) — recommended maximum of absorbed dose of radiation that a person or organ should receive in a specified period; for occupationally exposed persons, the MPD is 5 rem per year or 0.1 R per week; for occasionally exposed persons, the MPD is 0.5 rem per year or 0.01 R per week.

Magnetic resonance imaging (MRI) — technique of visualizing the body's soft tissues by applying an external magnetic field that makes it possible to distinguish hydrogen atoms in various environments.

Myelography — technique that combines radiography with fluoroscopy to evaluate the spinal subarachnoid space; after injection of an iodinated contrast medium into the subarachnoid space through a lumbar puncture, fluoroscopic images of the spine are taken.

Nidus — point of origin of a mass.

Oblique — slanting; a direction between horizontal and perpendicular; in radiology, a projection taken on a slant.

Opacification — process of rendering organs or body tissues whiter or brighter than surrounding tissue or adjacent structures on diagnostic-imaging film; achieved by using a contrast medium, which blocks penetration of X-rays.

Perfusion scan — nuclear-medicine study that produces a visual image of the blood flow and function of a specific anatomic structure after I.V. injection of a radioisotope; the radioisotope particles become lodged in the microcirculation of the structure under study, permitting their detection as light on a scanner; absence or paucity of these particles indicates poor perfusion.

Percutaneous transhepatic cholangiography (PTC) — fluoroscopic examination of the biliary ducts after injection of an iodinated contrast medium.

Percutaneous transluminal angioplasty (PTA) — procedure in which a narrowing in a blood vessel is opened; a balloon-tipped catheter is inserted through the skin and through the lumen of the vessel to the site of the narrowing; there, the balloon is inflated, flattening plaque against the vessel wall.

Photoelectric effect (absorption) — low-level energy produced when X-rays react with atoms of the body.

Piriform — pear-shaped.

Posteroanterior (PA) — from back to front; for example, a PA chest projection.

Radiation absorbed dose (rad) — basic unit for measuring an absorbed dose of ionizing radiation.

Radioisotope — radioactive isotope of an element used for the diagnosis or treatment of diseases and disorders.

Radiolucent — partly or wholly penetrable by X-rays; radiolucent areas are less dense than surrounding structures and appear black or dark on film; the lungs, for example, appear dark or black because air is radiolucent.

Radionuclide — a radioactive nuclide; a nuclide that disintegrates with the emission of electromagnetic radiations.

Radiopaque — not penetrable by X-rays; radiopaque areas, such as bones, appear white or light on X-ray because they're denser than surrounding structures; the opposite of radiolucent.

Radiopharmaceutical agent — radioactive chemical or pharmaceutical used in diagnosing or treating diseases and disorders; for example, radioactive substances injected I.V. for a nuclear medicine scan.

Radiosensitivity — property of being sensitive to radiation; some types of tissue and tumors are more radiosensitive than others.

Radiotracer — radioisotope injected into the body that can be seen on a nuclear-medicine scanner; as the radiotracer passes through and is metabolized by body structures, the function of the structures can be evaluated.

Roentgen (R) — in radiology, the unit of the emitted radiation dose.

Roentgen equivalent man (rem) — amount of ionizing radiation that has the same biological effect of 1 radiation absorbed dose of X-ray.

Sagittal — of or pertaining to an imaginary line extending from the front to the back in the midline of the body or a part of the body; sagittal X-ray images are of vertical slices viewed from right to left.

Scatter — deflection of X-rays or sound waves from the body.

Seldinger technique — technique used in angiography and some other procedures to insert a catheter into a hollow lumen or structure, such as a blood vessel; a needle is placed in the vessel, a guidewire is passed through the needle, and the catheter is advanced over the wire.

Sentinel loop — prominent distended loop of small intestine near the pancreas seen on plain films of the abdomen in some inflammatory pancreatic disorders.

Shadowing — radiographic phenomenon that occurs when a structure interrupts waves, resulting in diminished or absent echoes that obscure the image behind the structure; for example, gallstones, vertebrae, and air in the bowel may cast shadows and obscure structures.

Shield device — lead barrier used to protect a person from radiation.

Sievert (Sv) — measurement of the biological effect of radiation; international unit of radiation absorbed dose equivalent (1 Sv equals 100 rem).

Silhouette sign — phenomenon that occurs when an area of increased density, such as from an abnormality, hides a normal border of an adjacent structure; for example, a silhouette sign occurs when a border of the heart is obscured by fluid in an adjacent lung area.

Single-photon emission computed tomography (SPECT) — tomographic technique used to study blood metabolism. A radionuclide is injected I.V. and detected by a conventional scintillation camera or a rotating camera system; a computer reconstructs a three-dimensional image from the series of two-dimensional images produced.

Shuntogram — X-ray of a shunt taken as contrast medium is instilled.

Sonolucent — in ultrasonography, the property of allowing free penetration of ultrasound waves without reflecting them back to their source. Sonolucent areas appear dark or black on film.

Stent — slender, rod-like device used to support a vessel or other tubular structure or to establish or maintain its patency. The stent is mounted on a balloon-tipped catheter; when the balloon is inflated, the stent expands and adheres to the walls of the narrowed structure, bracing it open.

Thallium imaging — technique in which a radioisotope, thallium-201, is injected I.V. to evaluate myocardial blood flow and myocardial cell status; the isotope enters healthy tissue quickly; areas with poor blood flow and ischemic cells fail to take up the isotope and appear as cold spots on a scan.

Thermoluminescent dosimeters — devices worn by radiology personnel to measure radiation exposure.

Through transmission — in ultrasonography, free penetration of fluid by a beam of sound, which is then reflected back to the transducer off the structure behind the fluid collection; one of the criteria needed to define a cyst on ultrasound.

Transcranial Doppler ultrasonography — Doppler technique used to monitor blood-flow changes and emboli in intracranial vessels; the transducer, positioned at the temporal region of the patient's head, transmits pulses of high-frequency sound waves, which are reflected back to the transducer by red blood cells moving in the vessel being studied. Reflected sound waves are processed electronically into an audible signal and a waveform display on a monitor that provides information about blood flow and other diagnostic parameters.

Transesophageal endocardiography — ultrasonographic technique in which a transducer is guided into the esophagus to view the heart through the esophageal wall; eliminates interference from chest wall muscles, adipose tissue, air, and bony structures and allows a clearer view of the heart.

Transjugular intrahepatic portocaval systemic shunt (TIPS) — palliative procedure performed under fluoroscopic guidance to relieve portal hypertension or esophageal varices; a catheter is inserted into the internal jugular vein and advanced into the inferior vena cava, the hepatic vein, through the liver parenchyma and into the portal vein; a stent is then inserted to maintain this artificial communication.

Urography — radiographic examination of the urinary system using contrast medium.

Venography — radiographic examination of the veins using contrast medium.

Ventriculography — radiographic examination of the ventricle of the brain or heart after injection of air or another contrast medium.

Voiding urethral cystography — radiographic examination of the bladder using contrast medium, performed as the patient urinates.

i refers to an illustration; t refers to a table

i refers to an illustration; t refers to a table

i refers to an illustration; t refers to a table

i refers to an illustration; t refers to a table

i refers to an illustration; t refers to a table